OUTDOOR PHYSIQUE

YOUR PORTABLE BODY TRANSFORMATION

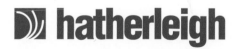

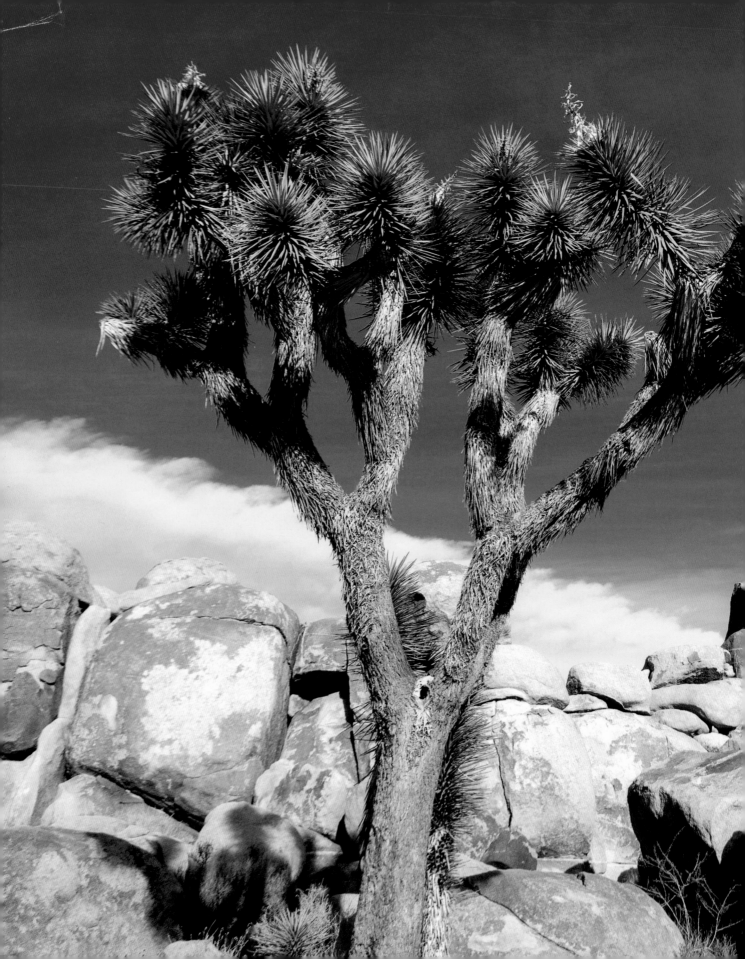

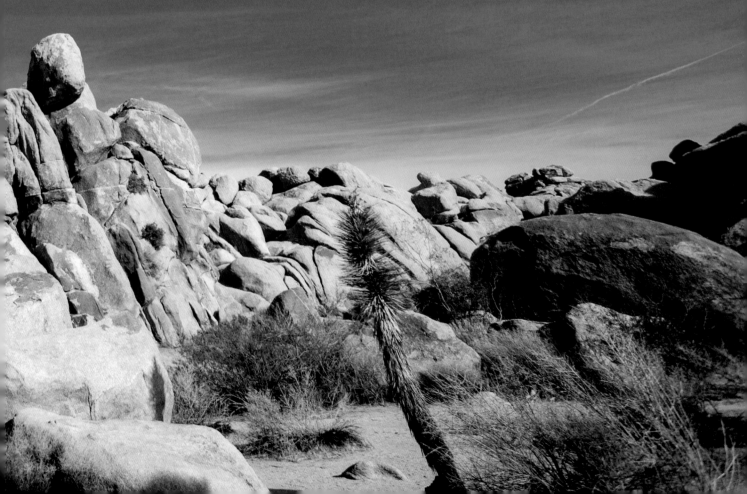

HOLLIS LANCE LIEBMAN

OUTDOOR PHYSIQUE

YOUR PORTABLE BODY TRANSFORMATION

Your health starts here! Workouts, nutrition, motivation, community…everything you need to build a better body from the inside out!

Visit us at www.getfitnow.com for videos, workouts, nutrition, recipes, community tips, and more!

OUTDOOR PHYSIQUE

Text Copyright © 2019 Liebman Holdings, LLC

Library of Congress Cataloging-in-Publication Data is available.
ISBN: 978-1-57826-833-7

Photography by Susan Sheridan Photography
Art Direction by Simon Murrell
Models: Hollis Lance Liebman and Daniela Schiller

Printed in the United States
10 9 8 7 6 5 4 3 2 1

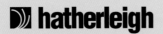

CONTENTS

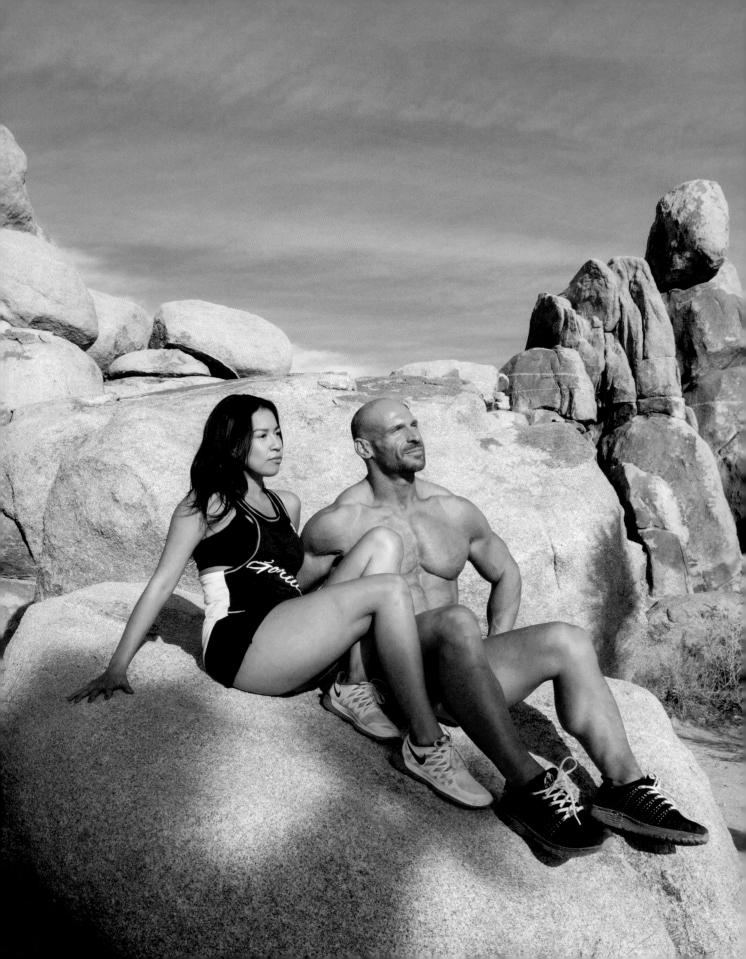

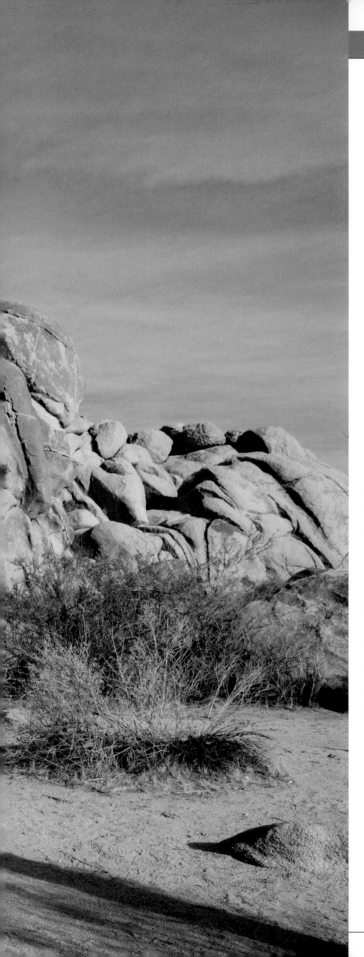

INTRODUCTION

"A select few are blessed with an intangible quality that allows them to perform at or near a level of perfection for a finite period, and then it's gone forever, never to return. Every sport carries its shining example. Some leave the sport they so love when the heart still says yes but the body has other plans. Some stay longer than they should. But they all leave at some point."

I wrote that paragraph a few years ago but never used it. And when formulating the initial ideas for this book, it came back to me. That was part of the answer. But what of the questions? Who is this book for, and for what purpose?

Some people just do not like the gym. Maybe you don't want to have to talk to anyone once there. Maybe you don't want to wait for the equipment, only to be faced with a sweat angel when it's your turn. Maybe you are tired of unsolicited tips on your form. Or you're tired of being leered at. Whatever the reason, it is okay not to like the gym. But it is not okay to let your goals and happiness wane as a result of that.

Outdoor Physique is for everyone. It is for anyone who cares not only how their body looks but also how it feels and performs. It is for anyone who has never quite felt comfortable in a gym. It is for those who can no longer lift the poundages they perhaps did when younger. It is for those who no longer wish to lift weights and are suffering with everyday aches and pains. And it is for those who would

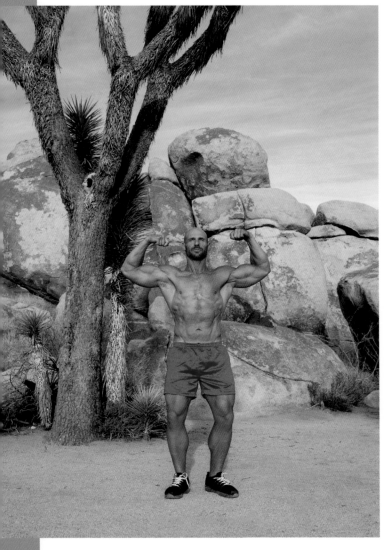

prefer ducking under a tree for shade instead of under the cold steel of a squat bar. Every at bat need not be a home run. Every exercise need not result in a new target set, a record, or a personal best. But every workout should be an attempt at empowering you. In short, *Outdoor Physique* is for those who are at another point in their journey and who wish to travel a different way along the path.

Different does not mean easier. It simply means by other methods. As we age, the importance we place on weights lifted or on chest or waist sizes diminishes as we focus more on getting around efficiently in life. You wake up one day, and instead of flexing your biceps, you place your hand on your lower back and wonder, "Will I be pain-free today?"

This book is for those who are interested in harnessing the near-limitless functional potential of their bodies. That does not mean there needs to be a step back in intensity or focus—or even in caring. It is designed for those of us who are less obsessed (albeit still mildly obsessed) with how we look and more concerned with how we feel and perform. After all, what good are a six-pack and well-developed arms if we struggle to change a tire or lift a gallon of paint off the floor? Disengaged from social media and its likes and approval, away from the gym and its artificial lighting and fancy machines, this book offers nature, movement, results, and—perhaps most importantly—happiness. Your happiness, in a way that feels organic to you.

Outdoor Physique is more than just a transformation book. You can call it a transition from one type of conventional training into a more open style, complementing actual movement. Call it going outside to play, just like we used to as kids. That is the thread running through this entire book: Put down your smartphone, and go and play outside.

MANDATORY UPLIFT

It is my sincere hope that *Outdoor Physique* is the book you've been waiting for. Having been a bodybuilder for most of my life, the cornerstone of my training was previously about building muscle for muscle's sake. I was confined to training muscles in isolation—that is, on "back day," my job was to work only my back and its intricate musculature. The result was strong, visually pleasing muscle that looked good on stage or on the beach but did little to help with taking my dogs on long walks around the neighborhood or

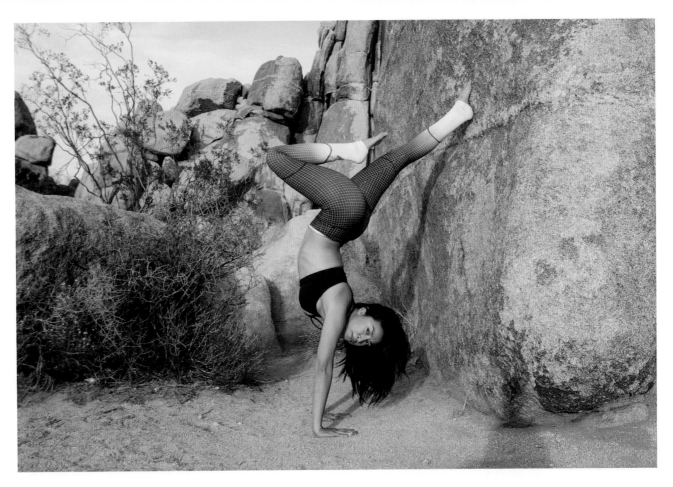

washing the floors in my home. In short, these muscles were all but useless in life.

The real world and its successful navigation require movement in which body parts work together—not in isolation, as in bodybuilding. On a daily basis we hardly consider which muscles we use, but when they all work together properly, tasks become far easier.

I have yet to be in a real-life situation where I'm pressing a heavy object directly off my chest as when doing a bench press, but many times I've had to remain in a mid-squat for prolonged periods while dealing with an issue in my basement crawl space. Bodybuilding didn't prepare me for it, but the training in this book did.

Of course, sometimes we have to change things even if we don't want to. Years of hammering away at muscles leaves few unscathed. I've had my share of battles in the gym, and I wouldn't trade those experiences, but one of the beautiful things about life is that it is ever changing. The human body—with its

infinite possibilities and the fact that we get to guide the ship—is indeed a beautiful thing. And the key here is that the ship must be continually steered.

We must keep on keeping on, because no one can run forever. Maximum force and intensity cannot be sustained indefinitely, or even for long, and why should they need to be? For it is truly about the journey. No workout program is ultimately about time parameters. Yes, a six-, eight- or 12-week plan might get someone to pick up the book and say, "I'm really gonna do it this time!" But it's about a life plan: Let's keep this thing—you—going and perhaps have some fun along the way.

This leads to what is perhaps the most important point: You are good enough as you are now. Many of us fervently believe that if we just *do this*, just *go here*, just *buy that*, just *lose the last bit of fat*, and so on, then we will have arrived, be good enough, be ready for the world. Of course, goals are important. But goals do not complete or define you. We must collectively disconnect from the "you're not good enough yet"

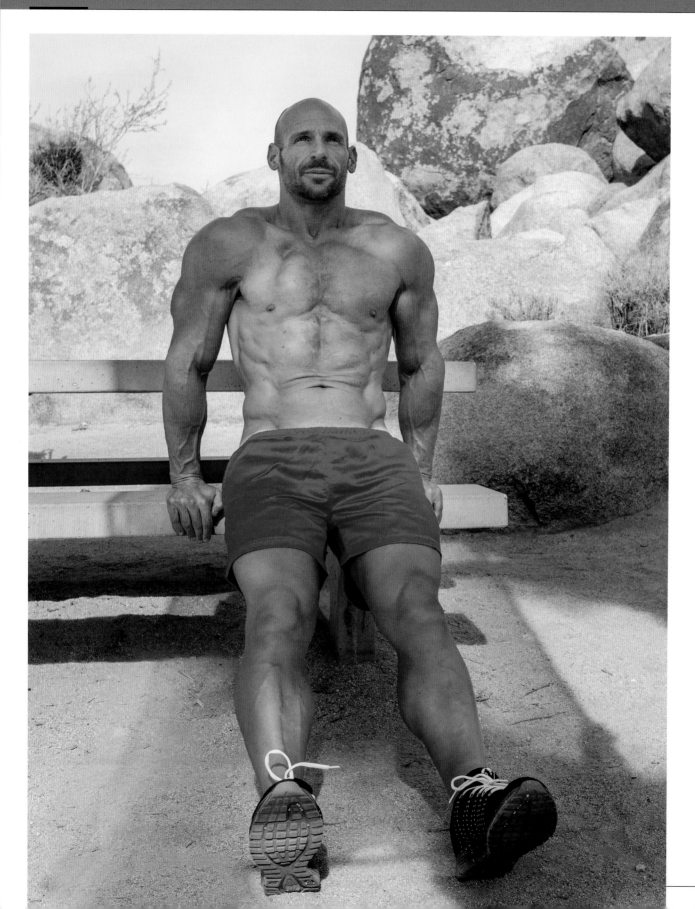

mind-set and shift our thinking toward "you're good to go now, and you're only going to get better."

Fat or thin, skinny or heavy, it doesn't matter. Those who use such labels are insecure themselves, trust me. Remember, we go to the gym (of whatever sort) so that we can look and feel good out of the gym. The damaging notion that we are not good enough yet, or that we will get to the gym just as soon as we lose this or gain that, is sheer nonsense.

KEEP 'EM SEPARATED

The challenge for this book was to create a portable plan based principally on using one's own bodyweight. Now, my friends, you are quite literally the gym. The workouts in this book can be performed just about anywhere that there's space and a surface.

Outdoor Physique is a metaphor for you: You are good as you are, and what you bring to the dance is more than adequate. This book is not about covering a zit or not showing up to school that day. This book is about the show goes on 24/7, rain or shine. We do this not for validation but for ourselves. This book is about being as present during your set as you are in your surroundings—in this book, that was the stunning Joshua Tree National Park, which is almost like a character itself in this story. The place of schooling can often be as important as the schooling itself.

This is not a fad book; it is an evolutionary book. While a bright-eyed, often youthful newbie picks up his or her first fitness magazine, gets bitten by the iron bug, and focuses on massive arms or a huge bench press, their elder counterpart has "graduated" to more personal and relevant needs, such as good health and movement. Just as once we were all pushed on a swing, we are now at the point of pushing someone else. We have evolved to the next level.

I grew up in the gym. My introduction to real exercise was on Nautilus machines, so I learned how to work and control my muscles through predetermined pathways of motion. Soon after, I discovered the rusty, clanking free weights in an old gym, and I fell in love. There was a direct correlation between how much effort I put in and the results I achieved.

But we get a little older and can't do what we used to. The weights seem to feel heavier. Little aches and pains precede the day's workout, starting straight after climbing out of bed. I woke up one day and truly realized it was now, for me, more important to move well than to move weights. Not lighter weights or less

intensity—I needed a new way, both mentally and physically. And *Outdoor Physique* was born.

The idea of working out in the open air, in a portable manner, without equipment; the idea of less pressure on the joints; the idea of free movement, strengthening real-world motion—this is what I explore these days, and I want to share it with you. *Outdoor Physique* is not a second-rate alternative to the gym, bodybuilding, or power-strength programs. It grew out of necessity. If you doubt its benefits, consider that my physique in these pages was forged largely from this program. Think it's just cosmetic? What I can do in my local park outstrips nearly anything I once did in the gym. And while I used to leave the gym with some sort of nagging pain, I now often leave the park wondering, "Where next?" *Outdoor Physique* is an all-in-one program. Fitness books tend to overpromise and underdeliver. They program you to race and pound and starve on weekdays, only to falter on the weekends. Every Monday is like confession, so you can simply start over after a weekend of binge eating. But this book is different, because everything is different—including you.

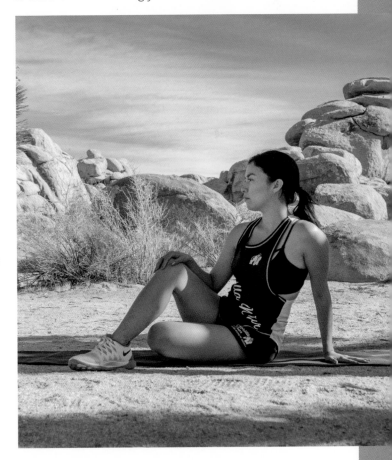

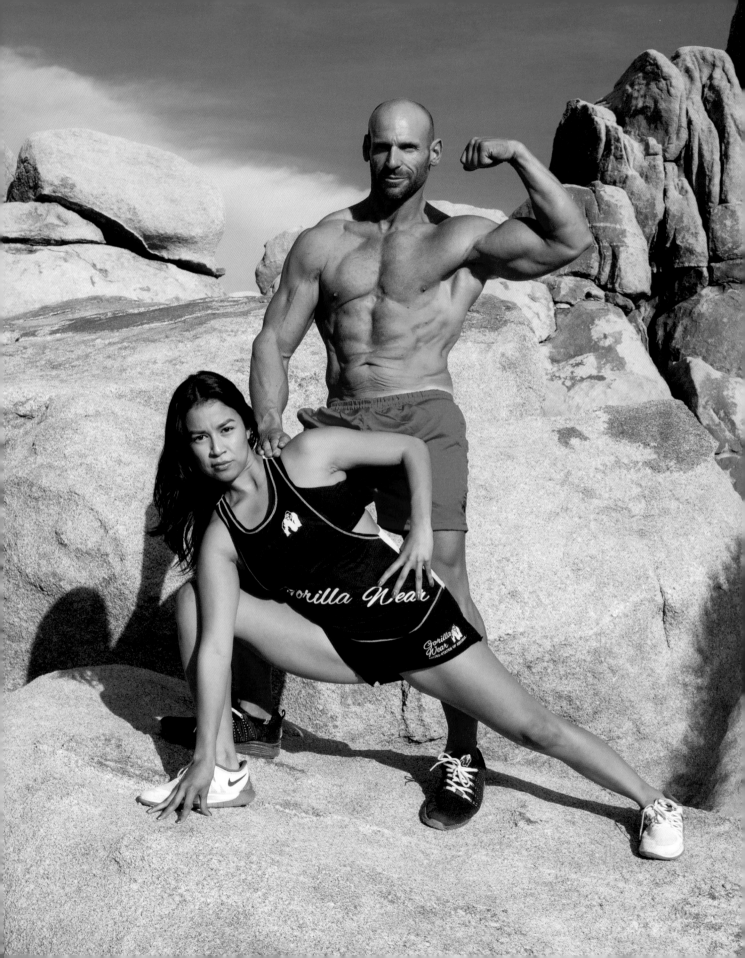

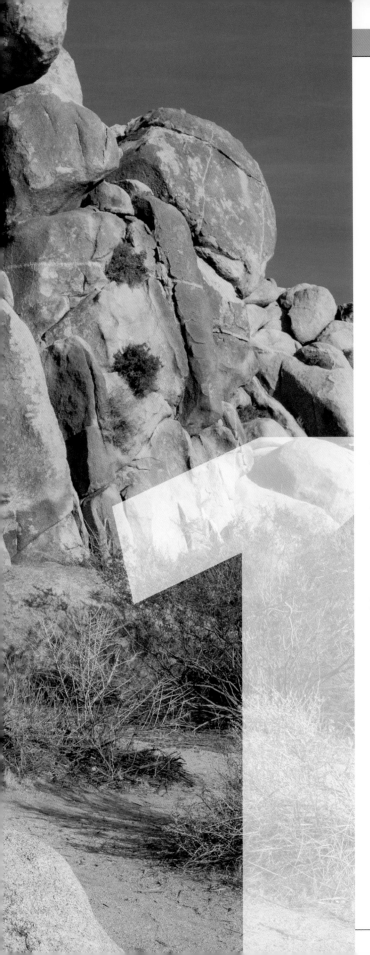

PLAN OVERVIEW

Generally speaking in the gym, it's up and down, inhale and exhale, stretch and squeeze. This repetitive pattern over a range of motion (often with machines) is the constant of gym life. Over and over again. Do X amount of reps, over X amount of sets, with X amount of weight, over X amount of time, and X amount of results can be yours. But real life is a bit different. We go forward and backward and side to side. We twist and shift and bend in myriad directions, and none of these actions are predetermined. We contort on the fly. Life is lived in 3D, not on limited and unmalleable, previously laid tracks.

The key consideration in designing and putting this book together was real-life movement. We are no longer limited to the negative, lowering portion or the explosive, upward positive extension of the arms on the bench press, because there is no bench press. Instead, there is real-world movement. The best training equipment is the human body, and results stem from movement. It's not enough to put out yet another bodyweight fitness book when there is already so much choice. What sets this book apart from the others is the planes of motion.

The three planes of motion are directions of movement that facilitate most of the body's mobility. The sagittal plane is an imaginary central line down the front of the human body, dividing it into left and right halves; motion along this plane includes forward and backward movement such as flexion (bending a limb or joint) and extension (lengthening a limb or joint). A line splitting the front and rear of the body gives the frontal plane; movements along this plane include lateral abduction (movement away from the midline of the body) and adduction (movement toward the midline of the body) utilizing the arms and legs. And a line drawn at roughly waist level is the transverse plane; this gives a twisting motion.

Generally, each exercise in this book is specific to one plane of movement and multiple muscles working along that plane. To complement the bodyweight movements and non-weighted resistance theme throughout, yoga and boxing have been added in.

PROGRAM BREAKDOWN

Outdoor Physique: Your Portable Body Transformation holds firm to the belief that more is not better. Only better is better. These workouts are not intended to be performed every day; rather, they should be carried out in levels ranging from three to four workout days per week. And because this is not another 12-week

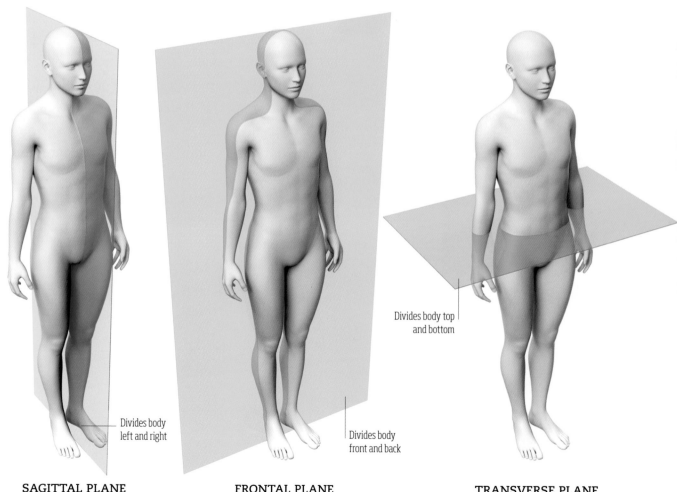

Divides body
left and right

Divides body
front and back

Divides body top
and bottom

SAGITTAL PLANE   FRONTAL PLANE   TRANSVERSE PLANE transformation program, you may rest and repeat ad infinitum. In a further departure from the other books in my series, this isn't for 12 weeks—it's for life.

This is a book about an ongoing lifestyle. We are not rushing or cramming to prepare for an upcoming event; we are *in* the event: life. *Outdoor Physique* can be practiced freely all year round wherever you are, indoors or out. And the goal is you getting back to greater living. Someone else has a greater bench press or more ripped arms or better abs? Great—more power to them. For competition is out, and self-reflection and empowerment are in.

While there are three phases of progression, once you reach the end, the sky is the limit. Phases 1 and 2 each last four weeks and simply build on one another. But Phase 3 is your life program, and it will enrich you time and time again in numerous ways.

A traditional bodybuilding program outlines a progressive program in which one or two muscle groups are worked once per week. Great, terrific, and effective, yes. But you're here because you want more and different. It's no longer about aesthetics; it's about functioning well and moving freely and with ease.

Outdoor Physique focuses on performance, on teamwork, on multiple muscle groups working together to steer the ship in the most effective way. To some degree, all of the major muscles will be worked in each workout in the book, because we are building functionality for performing a task or fulfilling a duty.

BODYWEIGHT BENEFITS

"Wait a minute," I hear you say. "You want me to give up my gym membership and my free weights to work out in the middle of nowhere?" Not exactly. Bodyweight workouts were around long before resistance exercise, and those ancient physiques were nothing to scoff at, so it's worth taking a closer look into what you've been missing.

While weight training consists largely of isolating specific muscles, bodyweight exercises can work many at once for a truly synergistic approach. Bodyweight exercises are safer, generally, over time than their weight-bearing counterpart, which can stress the joints. Even if you're totally pain-free, weight training sometimes gets boring, and bodyweight exercises can breathe new life into your routine. Actually, the word "routine" should be removed from the bodyweight-exercise practitioner's vocabulary, since making yourself your own gym is anything but routine.

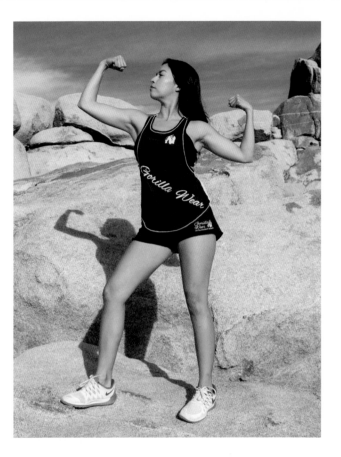

Lastly, the myth that push-ups, dips, and squats are the mainstay of bodyweight training and lack variants couldn't be further from the truth. With a mere angle change or slight body shift, you can transition almost effortlessly from one exercise to another. There are variants galore. The only limit is your imagination.

An important distinction here versus a traditional bodybuilding routine is that we are not trying to break down a muscle fully during a given workout. We are trying to improve its performance. In bodybuilding, let's say you completed a bench press max with 100 pounds for six reps. By definition, on the next chest workout the goal is to hit 100 pounds for seven to eight reps, and onward and upward. In *Outdoor Physique*, we do not attempt to lift more weight because you *are* the weight, or resistance, but we attempt to hold a pose for longer or perform more reps. This results in greater performance and conditioning, not necessarily the greater muscle circumference or density that one would see with conventional resistance training. It's like the difference between James Bond and the Hulk.

PICTURE THIS

If you've read some of my other books, you'll know I am not a numbers guy—that is, I don't need a number on a scale to tell me where someone is physically. The mirror, the photograph, and how your clothes fit tell me a lot more about your current shape and condition. But not even they reveal true ability, such as how well you perform forward/backward movements, side-to-side movements, and turning movements.

While improved performance is the main consideration of this book, it's also about bettering your insides, as well as your outside. And since nutrition has a direct effect not just on how you look and feel but also on how you perform, our aim is to improve your physique, both in performance and aesthetics.

Therefore, though there is no end to this program (as well there shouldn't be), I firmly believe in taking progress photographs of all four sides of the body. You can then refer back to them whenever you want

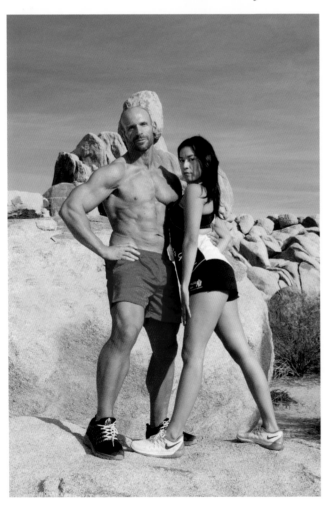

positive reinforcement, motivation, or a virtual pat on the back. Pictures will show you where you were, whereas your workload performance and, more importantly, your life performance show you where you are. So, do take those before pictures—you'll thank yourself later!

Above all else, *Outdoor Physique* is designed to be a long-term, sustainable regimen giving lasting results. It is not a quick fix, a fad book, or a flavor-of-the-month program. On the contrary, bodyweight exercises take us back to the beginning. We tend to forget that we already have all we need. We're not born with an instruction manual for our body, but we are equipped with the skills to make it work at its best.

When I first began weight training at age 13, I wanted not only to boost my self-confidence and stand up to the bully, I also wanted a huge bench press and thick arms. Such results are generally achieved through a combination of power movements, isolation movements (to strengthen the stabilizer muscles), and lots of muscle-building food. Having good genetics doesn't hurt either.

Our muscles tend to be more pliable and more accepting of "hardcore training" when we are younger. As we age, though, we need to pay more attention to pre-workout, post-workout, mobility, and the overall recovery from a workout. It's like skipping your vegetables as a kid but finding that you need those green nutrients when you're a grown-up.

In *Outdoor Physique*, we concentrate on how effectively you can lift across all the planes of motion. This is accomplished by working multiple muscles and joints in unison to complete a given task or, in this case, repetitions. During squats, it's the hip and knee joints; for push-ups, it's the shoulders and elbows. Bodyweight exercises tie muscles together in a way that machines, with their predetermined exercise pathways, and even free weights simply do not.

Once you've worked through the whole program, you may take a week or two off and then simply pick it up again and continue. *Outdoor Physique* is not like other programs: It's not about speed and momentum in an effort to beat the clock. It's not about winning medals and beating others. It remains as it was in the other books in this series: about bettering you. As you progress, push yourself not by doing more exercises but by tackling the more challenging variants and for a longer time. Above all, though, always use good form and keep your muscles working together.

PHASE 1: WEEKS 1–4
BEGINNER TRAINING PROTOCOL

At its outset, the program works to get you accustomed to the planes of motion and how they correspond to real-world movement. It also aims to build up your cardiovascular base in order to handle multiple muscle groups working together. You will rotate three differing full-body workouts weekly, based on the three planes of motion: sagittal, frontal, and transverse. In addition, the following supplemental modality categories are included: warming up, with mobility exercises; cardio, represented by boxing; and cooling down, with yoga. The cardio boxing exercises follow your main workout to further enhance your aerobic capacity, as well as to boost your metabolism for optimal performance. The net effects are twofold: to build you up slowly for greater workloads, and to avoid burnout. Remember, this is a life program, not a three-month program. You will conclude each workout with a relaxing yoga cool-down.

MONDAY
Mobility Movements / Full-Body Workout A / Boxing / Yoga

TUESDAY
Off

WEDNESDAY
Mobility Movements / Full-Body Workout B / Boxing / Yoga

THURSDAY
Off

FRIDAY
Mobility Movements / Full-Body Workout C / Boxing / Yoga

SATURDAY
Off

SUNDAY
Off

PHASE 2: WEEKS 5–8
INTERMEDIATE TRAINING PROTOCOL

By now, it's a habit. You will be seeing great improvement in your cardio conditioning, muscle use, body strength, and ability. As well as adding a fourth weekly workout and cardio session to your routine, at this point the warm-ups (with an extra mobility movement) and workouts themselves also challenge and build on the previous phase. And you are still allowed to have weekends off!

MONDAY
Mobility Movements / Full-Body Workout A / Boxing / Yoga

TUESDAY
Mobility Movements / Full-Body Workout B / Boxing / Yoga

WEDNESDAY
Off

THURSDAY
Mobility Movements / Full-Body Workout C / Boxing / Yoga

FRIDAY
Mobility Movements / Full-Body Workout D / Boxing / Yoga

SATURDAY
Off

SUNDAY
Off

PHASE 3: WEEKS 9–12 AND BEYOND
ADVANCED TRAINING PROTOCOL

In the final phase of functional transformation, the four full-body workouts and boxing cardio remain intact but have been intensified by the addition of a fifth modality movement and second sagittal plane movement at the end of each block to give a "giant set"–that is, four exercises back to back. This phase will lead to your greatest transformation and will carry you well beyond your current levels.

MONDAY
Mobility Movements / Full-Body Workout A / Boxing / Yoga

TUESDAY
Mobility Movements / Full-Body Workout B / Boxing / Yoga

WEDNESDAY
Off

THURSDAY
Mobility Movements / Full-Body Workout C / Boxing / Yoga

FRIDAY
Mobility Movements / Full-Body Workout D / Boxing / Yoga

SATURDAY
Off

SUNDAY
Off

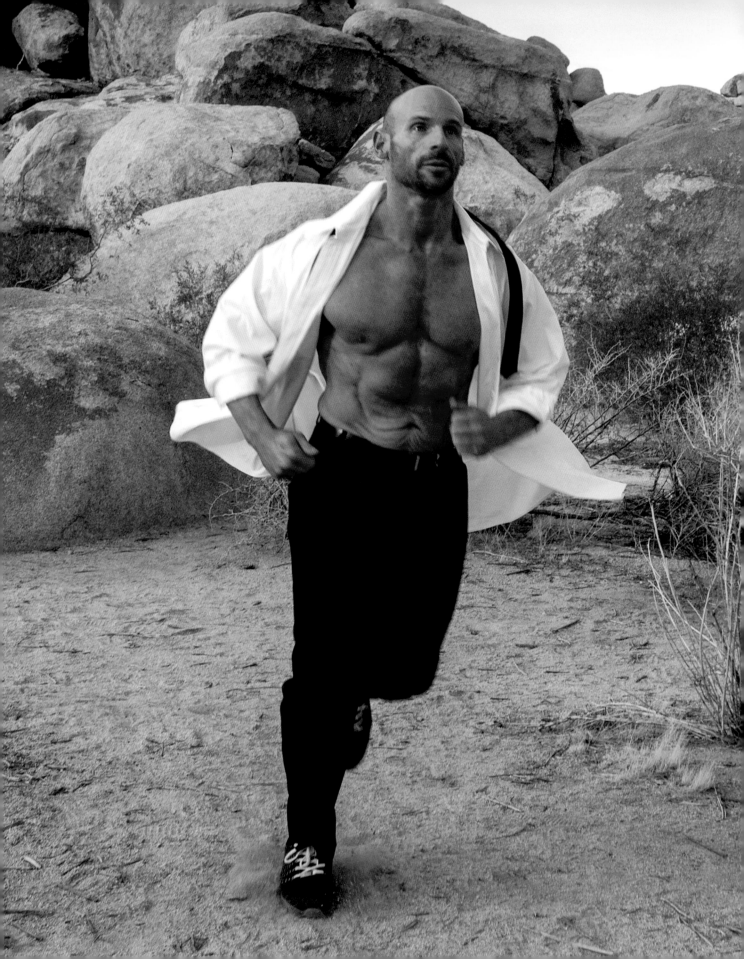

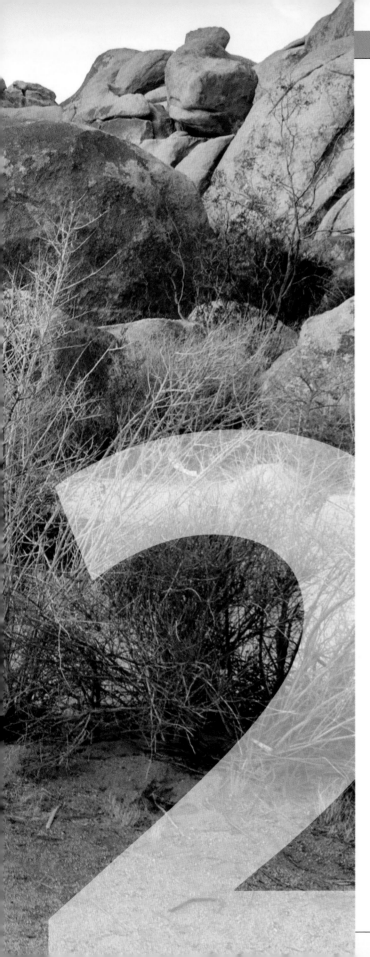

MYTH DEBUNKING AND LIFE OUTSIDE THE GYM

Back in our school days, we were taught to listen first and save any questions until after the teacher or speaker had finished. In this next chapter, I hope to address any of your queries or concerns about the program before you embark on it.

Q *Can bodyweight exercises really make me look as good as traditional weight training would?*

A It is certainly possible to attain a solid, ripped, rugged physique without resistance training. Other benefits of bodyweight exercises include less impact and stress on the joints, a greater focus on aerobic conditioning, and greater overall body performance. While you may not think bodyweight exercises will give you a 500-pound bench press or 20-inch arms, if you're holding this book, you probably want something different and of more importance to you.

Q *How soon will I start to see results?*

A When it comes to body performance and muscle quality, results depend on consistent and regular implementation of the program—not merely doing it for the sake of doing it, but doing it well. Coupled with proper nutrition, the workouts in this book should lead to noticeable results by the end of Phase 1. You should experience fewer muscle aches and pains, and some of the everyday hiccups of life will be reduced.

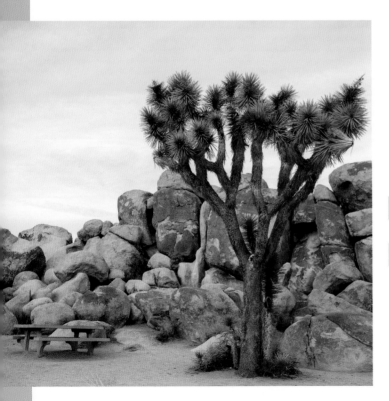

Q *Can I switch back to a more traditional routine if I'm so inclined?*

A It goes without saying that it's your body and your choice. Each book in the *Physique* series—this being the third and a departure from the other two—has its own unique program and protocol. That said, you can start and/or stay with any in the series. I would recommended, however, that you give *Outdoor Physique* a real shot. If you decide that you would prefer traditional bodybuilding results instead of all the benefits offered here, by all means make the switch. But you can come back to this program at any time, should you change your mind again. There are no rules, only suggestions. Even the exercises tend to follow a life movement or patterned pathway, as opposed to many rigid bodybuilding exercises, which are on a predetermined pathway.

Q *I've skimmed through the book, and I don't see any stretches. Where are the stretches?*

A Stretching is certainly important—so important that it has been covered in many other books, which is partially why it is not included here. Here, the stretching requirement has been filled by the inclusion of yoga. You may choose to stretch, of course, but it is strongly advised that you do so during or after exercise—never before. Your muscles must be warmed up and pliable before you begin stretching. Additionally, because most of the exercises in this book fall within the planes of motion, the idea is to stay loose and pliable throughout—that can be achieved by the inclusion of mobility movements.

Q *Regarding nutrition, why is there still an emphasis on protein? I'm not a bodybuilder.*

A Performance is fueled by carbohydrates and fats. These two macronutrients are merely energy, the fuel that goes in the tank. Protein is muscle. Protein is the engine. Without an engine, all the fuel in the world won't do much. While we are not here to construct the biggest, baddest engine, we are here to build a well-running, functionally sound engine—and to do so, we need engine parts.

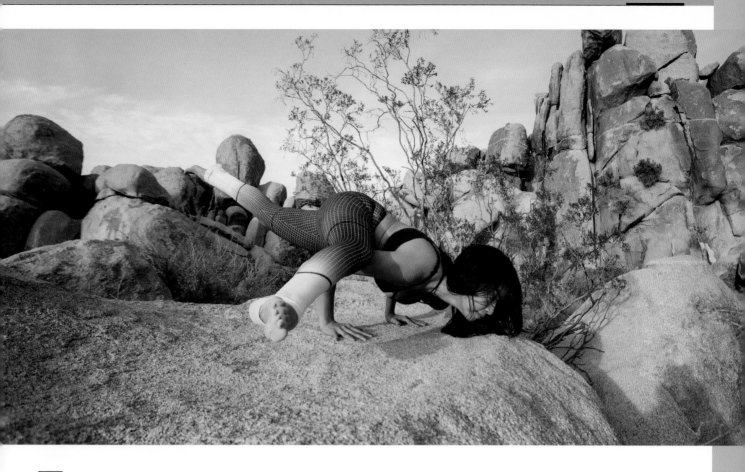

Q *I've got a previous injury. Is this program safe for me to follow?*

A Fitness is a personal journey that is different for everyone, but you should consult with your doctor first if you have any concerns about a current or previous injury. Having said that, life is risk. In traditional weight training, you may get pinned under a bar while bench pressing or nailed into the ground from squatting. But in bodyweight workouts, you are the resistance, and you can change the angle, speed, or pace at any time—or you can just stop. Listen to your body, and if something feels off or not quite right, don't do it. Pain-free training should always be of paramount importance.

Q *Can I do this with a partner?*

A Not only can *Outdoor Physique* be done with a partner—or even a group—but some of the exercises, such as the Ham Sandwich or Partner Push-Up, are designed to be done with a partner.

Working with a partner can help motivate you when you're not looking forward to working out or help on those days when some friendly competition can make things more fun.

Q *What do these words really mean, and does this book deliver them: functionality, aesthetics, longevity, and mobility?*

A Broadly speaking, these are the many benefits of bodyweight workouts. And yes, *Outdoor Physique* absolutely delivers them.

Functionality is about preparing the body to tackle the activities of your daily life.

Aesthetics refers to how your body looks in terms of muscularity. Genetics play a part, but you can enhance your body shape with exercise.

Longevity means your ability to perform well into your later years. Improved training, nutrition, and lifestyles have pushed the limits of human potential. No longer is 65 considered over the hill, spending the rest of your life in a comfortable armchair. People are living longer and enjoying a better quality of life into their later years.

Mobility relates to your body's ability to move comfortably and without incurring injury.

Q *What is the age limit for this program, and how far can you push your comfort zone?*

A If you're above ground and mobile, then there's no age limit. You can be pushed as far as you're willing and able to go, taking into account previous injuries or conditions. When I take on a new personal-training client, I don't have them fill out forms or bog them down with questions. All I need to know are their goals and any possible ailments, and we go from there.

Q *What exactly is overtraining, and is that possible here? I heard that doing push-ups every day is the best way to get better at doing them.*

A Overtraining is a state in which your muscle have not sufficiently recovered from previous workouts before tackling the next, due to a lack of rest and/or nutrition. It's something like a boxing match with no rest between rounds: You wouldn't be able to go very long or perform very well.

Training longer as opposed to better is usually what leads to overtraining, so the key is training smarter. If you were to attempt a max set of push-ups every day, by the third or fourth day you would feel the effects of the previous days' push-ups and would be unable to give your all. Instead, aim to perform them fewer times per week but to a higher standard. Think of it not as more mediocre food frequently, but better-quality food less often, leading to a much more desirable experience overall.

Q *Why can't I just stick to cardio? Doesn't that make me more functional?*

A Cardio exercise requires consistent motion for 20 minutes or longer, with the intention of raising the heart rate. For our purpose, the effect of cardio work is twofold: to improve metabolic efficacy—that is, the rate at which your body converts calories into energy—and to improve functional conditioning, or your ability

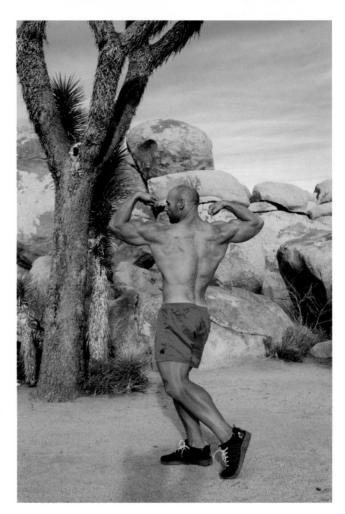

to move longer easier. Aerobic activity by itself is ineffective at improving your actual body composition. It doesn't build muscle. If you want to get lean and increase the strength of your muscles, you need to build muscle. Those reliant solely on cardio will retain a soft look to their bodies and be cheating themselves out of a body that can truly perform, not just in the long run but also in regards to strength.

Q *Can't I just keep it simple and stick to machines and cardio?*

A You could, but that's like shopping for shoes and ending up buying a shower curtain. Both are effective, but you came for one specific thing. Despite being good at building strength and improving your body composition, machines lack coordination, stability, and independent movement patterns. Also, many machines tend to start in the negative or downward position of an exercise, doing a movement that has no true real-life application.

Q *This program seems too broad. What if I want to focus on specific areas?*

A Spot reduction is the attempt to whittle fat away from one area, and it is myth—it doesn't work. When we burn fat, we burn it throughout the body, not from one particular section. Want to lose some fat off your abdomen? Losing fat there means you may also see a firming up of your arms, back, and more. Genetics also has an influence. In my family on my mother's side, we tend to store body fat first on our rear ends, and that seems to be the last place it comes off as well, regardless of how many squats and lunges I do. But by trusting in the process and not making rash decisions or skipping certain parts of the workouts, it will all fall into place.

Additionally, *Outdoor Physique* is effective because it is not an isolationist program. Because many muscles are working together, you will propel your body to a greater degree of efficacy, and fat-burning and strength-generating results.

Q *I'm a woman, and my needs are different than a man's. Is this book for me?*

A While males and females have different hormone distribution, the goals and means to attain those goals remain related. Both men and women respond in the same favorable way to training. Both sexes also have the same muscles. Women (generally) simply do not possess the genetics to become as muscular as men. And again, this is not a bodybuilding book—not that that should or would preclude you from picking one up and making some awesome changes possible. *Outdoor Physique* focuses on functional strength and beauty. Now, who doesn't want that?

Q *I need ever-changing intensity. How will this program continue to challenge me?*

A Nearly all the exercises in this book can be made easier or harder by just shifting your bodyweight

and changing angles. An arm or leg raised here, an altered position there, and an exercise that seemed easy becomes challenging once again. The only limit is your imagination. It's not about doing more; it's about doing it better.

Q *Abs, abs, abs! Are they covered in this program?*

A Your abs do much more than just draw eyes to them. They are responsible for contracting the trunk at the waistline, as well as keeping your body stabilized. And they are worked in just about every exercise you can think of. Think of them perhaps like the Wizard of Oz: not readily visible but there behind the scenes, making sure everything runs smoothly. Not only will you find

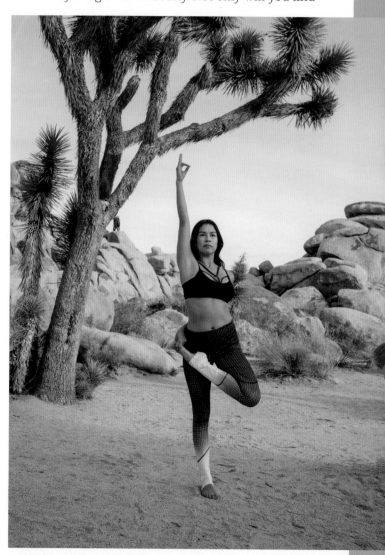

"direct" ab exercises such as the Medicine-Ball Chop in the program, you'll also find the abs indirectly worked during such movements as Shove-Offs. Try running through the program, and you'll see and feel your abs at work.

Q *Do I need to go to failure like in bodybuilding to produce results?*

A Absolute failure, as in a progressive overload in bodybuilding, is important for building bigger muscles. Otherwise, lift the same, look the same. But our goal here is not bigger muscles; it's better-functioning and stronger muscles. Failure in which one more rep is absolutely not possible is less important for our endeavors here than feeling the muscles working together. Also, we are after improved stability and coordination. Muscle groups working in harmony take the brunt of the workload away from any one muscle, thereby reducing the need for any

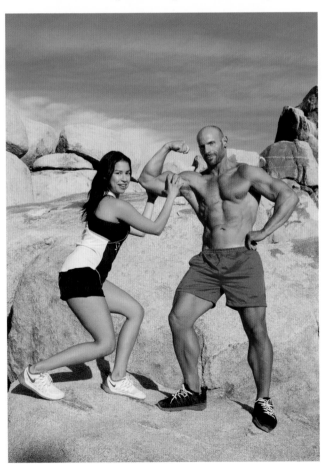

one muscle to be more developed than any other, as in bodybuilding. Complete each rep, exercise, and workout not in a rushed, get-it-over-with fashion but in a productive and flowing manner.

Q *Will bodyweight exercise help improve my posture?*

A Good posture aligns everything in the body, which is one of the added benefits of performing exercises using largely your own bodyweight. Not only are posture-improving exercises often easy to perform, but they also require very little equipment, if any. The key is having a strong core, which is put to the test during, say, Iron Crosses. Focusing on keeping your limbs long and your technique correct will help correct your posture.

Q *What is the difference between a full-body workout and a bodyweight workout?*

A A full-body workout session works most of the muscles in your body. You could also consider a full-body workout to be any that covers your chest, back, thighs, and hamstrings. Generally, a full-body workout is performed with resistance exercises. A sequence of barbell squats, bench presses, and triceps extensions would be a full-body workout.

A bodyweight workout follows similar lines in that multiple muscle groups are worked. The major difference, however, is that no weights are used; instead, one's own body is used as resistance. Squats, push-ups, and dips are examples of bodyweight exercises.

Q *Is bodyweight training safe or safer than weight training for a beginner?*

A Studies suggest that whether bodyweight or resistance exercise, the important factor is good form and good workout habits. Bodyweight training perhaps allows people to gauge more accurately the perfect resistance for them, eliminating the possibility of being pinned under a barbell during bench presses, for example. Given the choice, I'd suggest perfecting bodyweight exercises first and then moving onto resistance training.

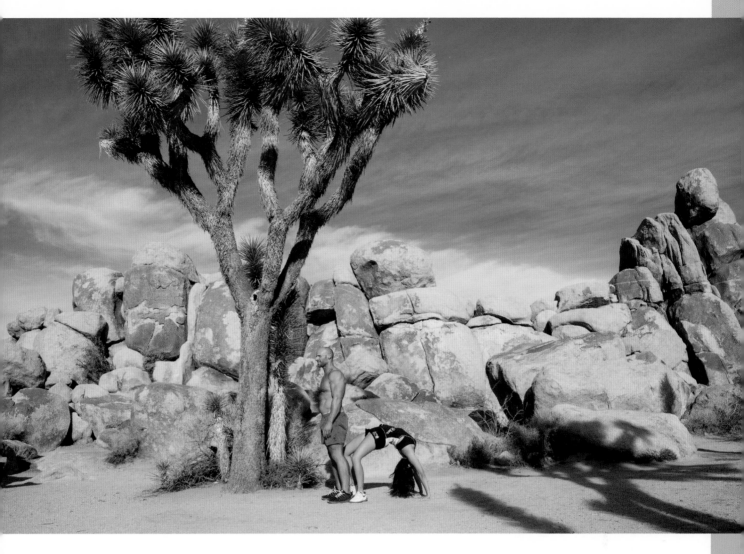

FAREWELL TO WEIGHTED ARMS

There's a scene at the end of the last *Lord of the Rings* movie, in which Frodo, still young in age, wants to travel with the elder folk and cross the waters to a new land. For many, *Outdoor Physique* is that next realm. A putting-down of the weights and picking up, literally, of yourself. This book is the next step in your own personal evolution.

Life is constant change. Many choose to stay within the confines of the weight room, with its cold steel and iron-wrought body. And that's fine. But others want more than that. In the process of bringing this book together, I chose to distance myself from the weight room and deliver functional and aesthetic results in a different way. Not because ego dictated it, but simply because the need is there.

As stated previously, for many the desire and ability to build the biggest arm muscles diminishes over time. Time and time again, I have seen the world's leading fitness competitors reach their peak and begin sliding down the placings. That's the hard reality of life. One former competitor severely blew out his knee at a photoshoot when he was encouraged to squat particularly heavy just a few weeks out from a judged event. Quickly his priorities changed to making sure he was able to walk again.

Also touched on earlier is the outdoor location as a character itself. That is the beauty of the portable workout: You get an experience training without excess equipment in the location of your choice— and you don't even have to wear a shirt.

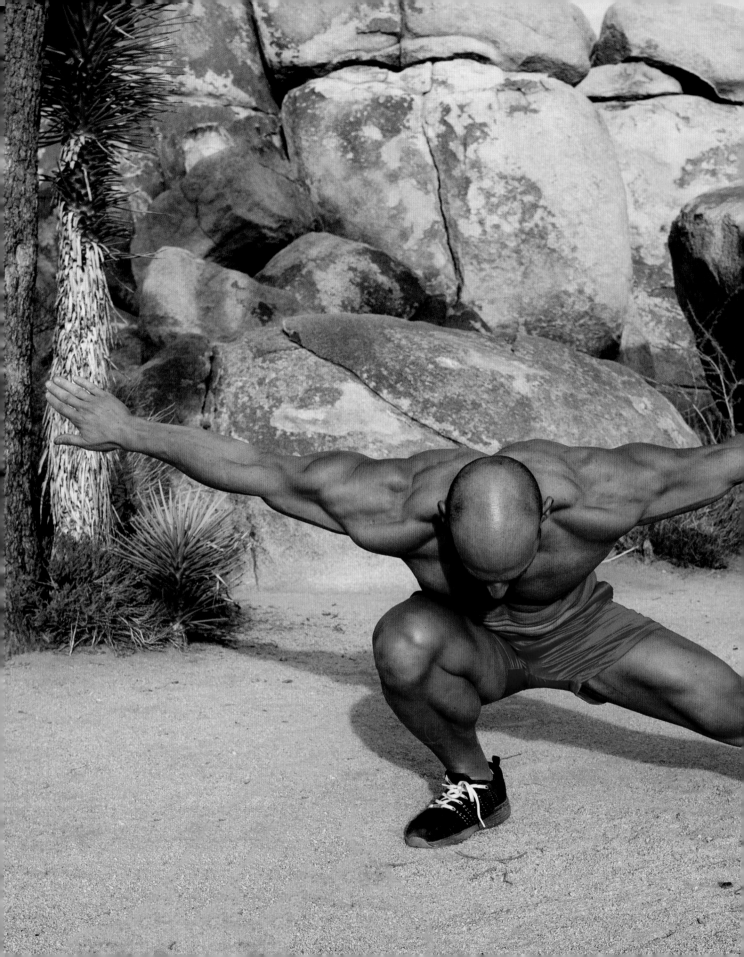

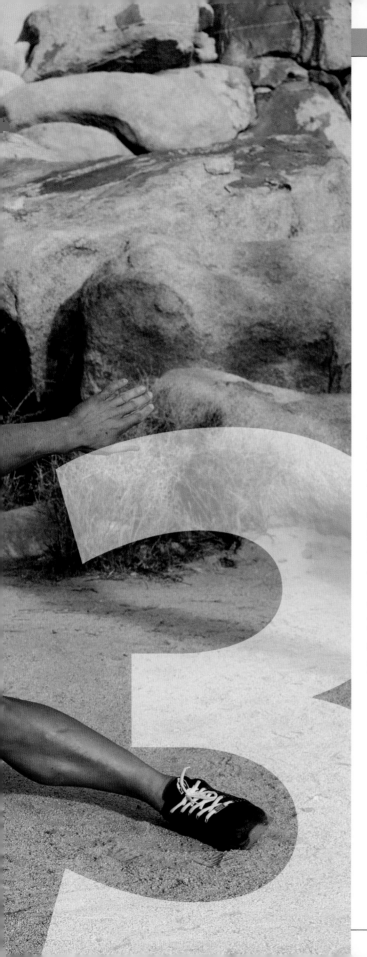

FOREVER MOTIVATED

Passion is the heartbeat of achievement. That's right. I thought of that one day while deciding what to post on my social-media platforms. And it's true: Without passion, sure, you can go through the motions for a period of time. You might even be able to accomplish something, but you can't give and produce something at your absolute best if you don't truly care. Even when you are paid for your efforts, it can sometimes be hard to give your best without having a vested interest.

On a personal note, prior to getting into shape for this project, I'd suffered a setback. But the thrill of creating this book was enough to get me back on track and excited. Since I was now a little older, with a few more battle scars than I was at the outset of the other two *Physique* books, the challenge was tough. One day, about three weeks before the photoshoot was to take place, a friend and I visited the gorgeous Joshua Tree location to take some test photos. And even at three weeks out, I simply wasn't ready. A real friend will say to you what was said to me that day: "In a tank top, you look great. But shirtless, you're not book-ready."

The comment stung. And then I went to work, and I delivered what was needed for this book. And I thanked my friend. Then, just like that, after the photoshoot, the ride was over. A feeling of depression set in, and someone told me this was common among marathon runners once they've run the big race. The daily routine was over and done; now what?

The "now what" is to focus on the next task. In this case, writing the book. Like Tarzan in the jungle, I now had the next vine to swing to. But I knew even that next stage would come to an end. So, the real trick is in keeping the momentum going.

The truth is, we can't always be passionate about what we do. Sometimes it is possible to do a job or task with integrity and then clock out. Every at bat need not be a home run, but we must at least get up and attempt to bat. You may no longer need to lift bone-crushing weights in the weight room, but you do need an outlet for your physical and mental self.

Of course we want outstanding results, but we also want realistic long-term results and a plan we can live with. When the shock of the new has passed, we have

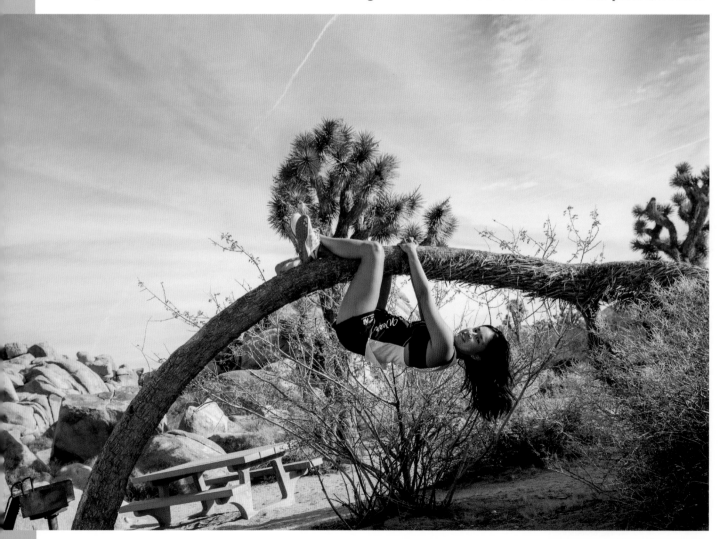

to work with what we've got. Passion gets us started, but we need something else to stay rooted in the game. If you can keep your physique permanently peaked, then kudos. But most of us are simply looking to keep the fire lit.

ACCELERANT

To excel, or not to excel—is that the question? I've noticed a lot of self-help books pump us up and get us ready to reenter the game called life: Put on a big smile, shoulders back, head high. But more often than not, things don't quite go to plan, and we end up feeling frustrated and dejected.

Instead of being laser-focused on seeking the gold medal, what if it was okay just to get the blue participation ribbon? What if more importance was placed on taking part rather than on winning? Failing is okay. It gives us experience.

In advance of the photography for this book, I did my usual social-media announcements (which keep me accountable), took unflattering before pictures, and marked "shoot day" on my calendar, along with workout notes on the interim dates. But then something happened that hadn't before: I just couldn't get into it. I couldn't even swing the bat, let alone hit the ball. Then I had a moment of clarity: I realized it was simply not yet the time to be "perfect."

As the months went on, I was able to put myself fully into something I believed in: the power of dreams, and the need to write the truth and help people. I also chose to walk before attempting to run. Before long, clothes that used to fit snugly were loose on me. Some of my friends said I looked skinny, but once my sweatshirt came off, I looked big, full, and ripped. The quest then became more than a book—it was about bettering my previous conditions. It was highly personal, and what started as trying to excel morphed into something more powerful: an accelerant.

What had been missing was a motivating factor, something that gets us excited about goals and dreams. Sometimes we just need to remember why we fell in love with something in the first place.

It's true to say my abs faded somewhat a few days after the shoot, once some cheat meals were reintroduced, and then it became about tangible sustainability: Let's look decent in jeans and a T-shirt and be able to function well on a daily basis. And that is the overriding goal and message here.

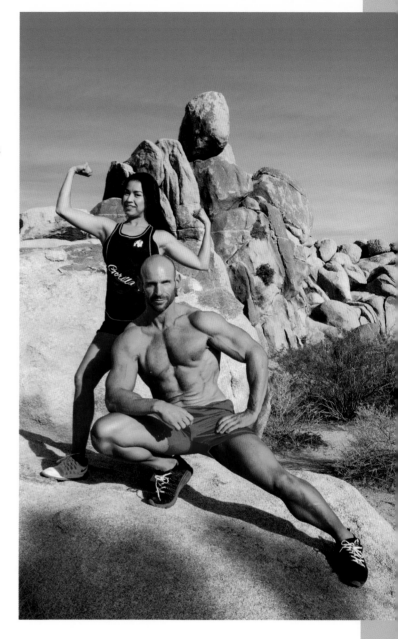

In some of my other books, I've focused on those who seem able to eat whatever they want and struggle to gain weight (*From Slight to Might*), those hell-bent on getting back to their previous bests (*Peak Physique*), and those wanting to stay close to the bull's-eye for the long haul (*Complete Physique*). But *Outdoor Physique*—in addition to helping, motivating, and stimulating—is for the individual who is looking for more.

Life is change. Nothing stands still forever. We grow older. So, the question is not about preventing aging; it's about managing to remain active as we age.

PROGRESSIVE PROGRAMMING

There are days when you wake up ready to take on the world, and there are days when you feel broken. We place so much pressure on ourselves to succeed that anything less than an annihilating victory is often considered a failure.

But it's okay sometimes not to smile. It's okay to jab instead of uppercut. It's okay sometimes not to feel your best or to feel in a cloud. We are allowed to go through the not-so-desirable emotions to get to the good stuff—indeed, sometimes it's necessary. You have to peel away the rind to get to the sweet fruit.

Progressive programming is a mind-set that sometimes stumbles and fumbles and sidesteps but never ever retreats. Fitness is not a finite journey; it is a malleable, ongoing existence that becomes as much a part of our lives as brushing our teeth.

When we can look past the daily grind, when we can overcome the feelings of resistance and instead choose persistence, that is when we are utilizing progressive programming. My progressive programming for the photography in this book was accomplished with small goals in training, nutrition, and recuperation. Though there were days I didn't want to work out or I wanted to eat sweets, I kept progressing. I combed the food aisles and stocked my cart with forbidden treats to keep at home until after the photoshoot, and I found this was helpful in fortifying me for success. I felt a power in it, knowing that I could reward myself after the mission was concluded. And of course after indulging myself, I returned to having a junk meal only every few days.

THE UNLIMITED SELF

There was a segment on an episode of *Mister Rogers' Neighborhood* when I was a child that has always stayed with me. The then NFL superstar Lynn Swann was a guest on the show. Aside from his numerous football accolades, Lynn was a practitioner of ballet, which he credited with helping him on the field. He spoke passionately on the subject, and for me the takeaway was never to let someone compartmentalize you. Set your own limits, and define your own self.

For things to work well, they need to be made well. Today, a lot of technology products are not built to last. They serve a function for a finite period of time, and then we buy a replacement or an upgrade. We can't throw away our bodies—but we can give them some sort of upgrade. If we take the time to lay down

a strong foundation, we can build a sturdy structure on top of it. When we don't rush our workouts and are present within them, we can communicate better with our bodies and achieve results more quickly.

The ever-changing image in the mirror and the desire to navigate through life easily are the sources of your consistent motivation. During my preparation for the photos in this book, I often said it would be the last photoshoot with me modeling. That may or may not turn out to be true, but I needed to believe it at the time so I could give my all to the prep and create an inspiring result. The photoshoot ended, of course, but that doesn't mean the lifestyle did. I still love to train and eat clean, and I also really love those cheat

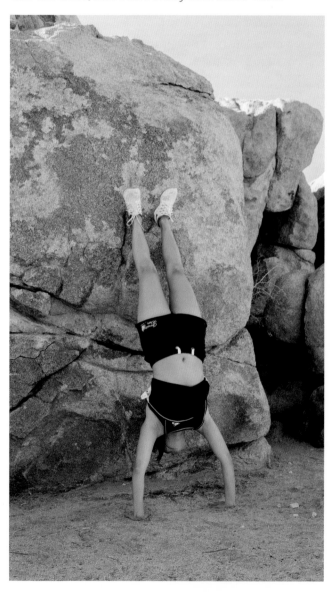

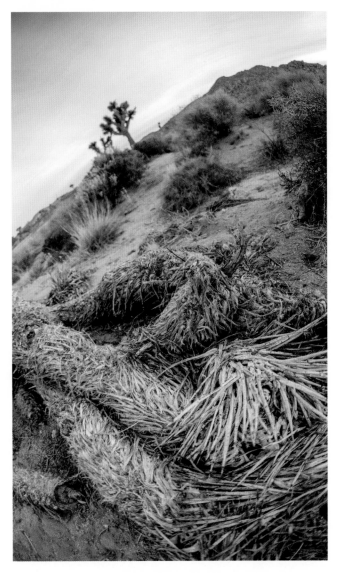

RELAXED MOTIVATION

There are certain truths and beliefs that will help you stick with your program for a lifetime and not just 12 weeks or so. Trust in progress, not perfection. If you're obsessed with perfection, you put too much pressure on yourself and you will create a goal that, even if achieved, is impossible to maintain. This doesn't mean you should begin without a plan; just reduce the pressure and increase the enjoyment.

Fitness is a personal journey. You're the one doing the exercises day in and day out and making the food choices—but sometimes it's good to partner up. When you're having a tough day or are lacking motivation, partnering up can make all the difference.

Sometimes the only barrier between getting it done and not is how many people know of the plan. Making it public often makes it stick. Posting a flattering (or unflattering) picture on social media and announcing your goals publicly can draw people in. Likes and comments can help keep us focused.

Make it a promise, and keep it unbreakable. But remember that it's okay to miss a workout here and there or switch workout days. But if you do trade days, be sure to keep it honest and keep your word.

INSTINCTIVE GAINS

When I first joined a gym, it became my daily vacation and salvation. But I knew I was there for one purpose: to improve my physique. As in everything in life, there is always someone better than you; this is a good thing, for it can and should help motivate you.

There was this enormous man at the gym, with gigantic tree-trunk legs. But what I routinely witnessed motivated me because I knew it was what not to do. He would walk out of the squat rack with 500 pounds across his trapezius, then bend his knees a few inches and stand back up, huffing and puffing, before doing it again. That's no squat! I found it laughable and annoying at the same time, and I used it to motivate me.

I knew that, for a squat to be effective, one had to squat low enough for the thighs to be parallel to the ground and then push back up through the heels, not the toes. I would use a weight I could control and I did this routinely, until my thighs grew. I've always believed, if you're going to duck under a bar, it's best to do it correctly. And the other thing I learned was this: You have to earn it, every day. Whether in the gym, outside, or even at your writing desk, you have to keep earning it.

meals—but looking, feeling, and functioning well year-round is something to aspire to.

Animals stretch upon waking because that is what they do. You work out and follow a clean lifestyle because that is what you do. This program is, by virtue of being in your hands right now, the next logical progression, whether you are coming to physical exercise for the first time or are simply looking for a change from weights.

Life is constant reinvention. It is up to you to pick the path that gives you the most pleasure. And one of the exciting things about life is how priorities change. When we can look in the mirror and still feel passionate, still feel as if the road continues, still want to better ourselves in diverse ways, life can be a joy.

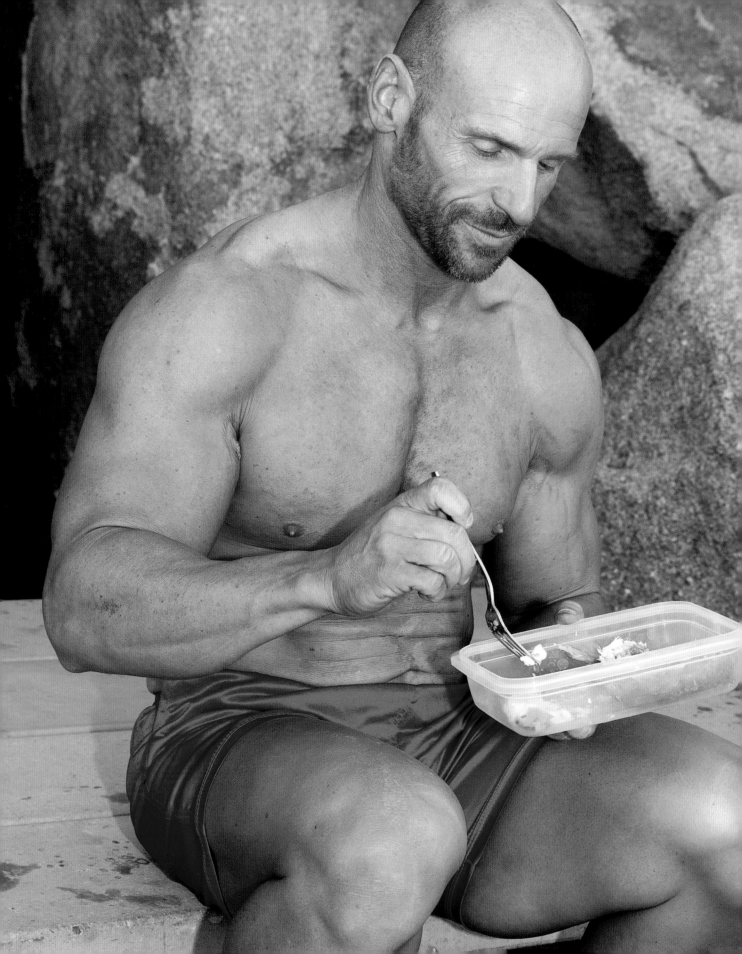

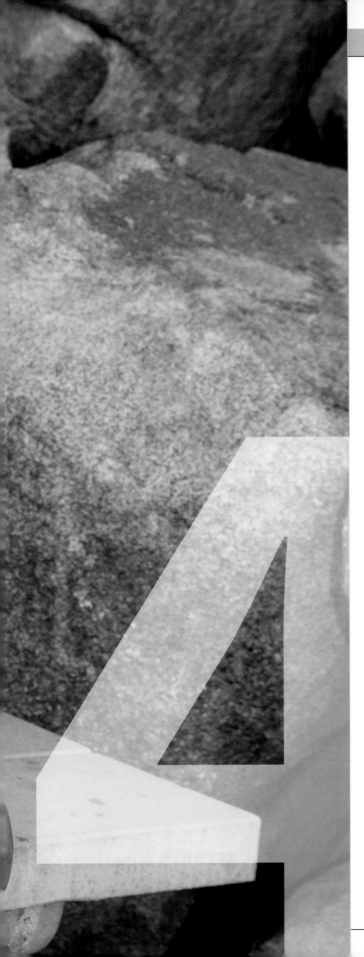

THE FUEL

As far as diet—or as I like to call it, fuel—and lifestyle go, *Outdoor Physique* offers a functional fitness program to power you and advice on functional eating to sustain you. And by functional, I mean catering not to your emotional needs but to your conscious ones, to help you move and live better.

There are plenty of books that delve deeply into the nutritional requirements of bodybuilding—that is, for attaining maximal lean muscle with minimal body fat. But the way of eating discussed in this book is less about aesthetics and more about getting good marks on your annual health checkup. *Outdoor Physique* is about eating for sustenance and performance first, with definition and aesthetics to follow. What good are big arms if they don't help you get through life?

You do not have to be miserable or suffer to create a body that not only looks good but performs even better. Real, unprocessed food will power you through your workouts and empower you through life. Eat less man-made, manipulated food, and you will have a far more sustained level of energy.

There are three major macronutrients in food: proteins, carbohydrates, and fats. Carbs and fats are simply energy, used by your body to keep you powered during physical and mental tasks. Protein, on the other hand, is what we are composed of. Protein is muscle,

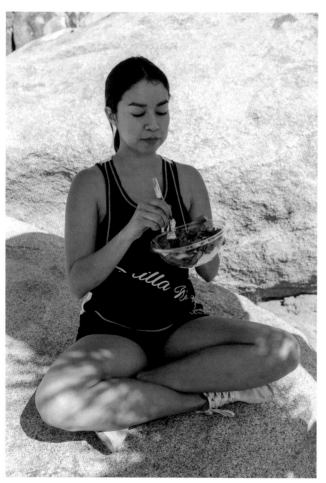

and muscle is what *does* the tasks. To utilize, build, and preserve muscle, we must consume protein.

Through all the fads, books, products, and types of diets, one consistent truth is that "whole foods" produce whole results. Vegetables, fruits, nuts, seeds, grains, eggs, fish, and lean meats should be the cornerstone of your daily consumption.

NEED TO KNOW

If you've read this far, it's not theory you're after, it's performance. Just what exactly needs to go under the hood to make this engine of yours run well? And how can you apply this to your busy life?

Certain things must be cut or changed if you want results. First, the word "diet" needs to be reconfigured, because this should be a permanent lifestyle change, not a temporary one. Second, *Outdoor Physique* is not for those who want to be skinny; it is for those who want to be lean and functional. Eating need not be driven by hunger; it can be driven by performance. A meal is a pit stop in preparation for activity.

The best meal plans are those based around good, nutritious fuel taken at multiple pit stops throughout the day. Think of these feeding times as evenly spaced supports holding up a bridge. When you give the body what it needs, it will spare the muscle tissue and instead utilize fat as fuel.

As a rule of thumb, about a third of your meal plate should be from a lean protein source. Chicken and turkey breast, fish, eggs, and lean meats such as top round or flank steak and buffalo are excellent sources of protein. Half the remaining portion should be composed of a complex carbohydrate to provide sustained energy—so, brown or white rice, yams, potatoes, oatmeal, quinoa, or beans, for example—with the remaining portion being a fibrous carb for digestion, such as greens or vegetables.

THE GOOD, THE FAT, AND THE UGLY

For a while, low-fat diets were all the rage, because "fat must be what's making me fat, right?" But when fat was removed from meals, sugar was often added in to make the food palatable. And these meals left people feeling weak and tired and craving more food. But with all that extra sugar, people were gaining weight—and when I say weight, I mean fat.

Fat is our friend, and its inclusion in your daily diet will not only help you lose fat, it will also help your performance. By including unsaturated fats in the form of seeds and nuts, healthy oils, and fish, you will sate your hunger and provide your body with good, sustainable energy.

I took in more fats than usual while preparing for this book for two reasons: to power my training and to come in leaner. The results speak for themselves. The key is to strive for balance, not perfection.

THE GEARS OF APPLICATION

The first gear is to invest in yourself by eating properly. It takes very little time to grill some chicken, microwave some potatoes, and put a salad together. Then you can put it in Tupperware to take with you for the day. It takes mere minutes to fortify yourself for success.

The second gear is to take imperfect action. Don't worry about painstakingly measuring everything out. Through the years, experience has taught me what looks about the right portion size for my nutritional intake. Remember, this is a lifestyle, and the longer you do it, the easier it will be.

The third gear is to stop comparing yourself to others. This is about you. If you look at someone you wish to emulate, that's fine—it's a good thing. But if you compare yourself to them and try to fill in where you see yourself coming up short, that's counterproductive. If someone is eating dry tuna fish and oatmeal, don't feel bad that you're not eating as clean. Equally, don't feel tempted into treating yourself just because someone is biting into a triple-stacked bacon cheeseburger. Carve your own path.

The fourth gear is to shift gears. You must walk before you can skip. Don't become overwhelmed; become empowered. "I can't eat all that food," you may be thinking, but as your workouts increase in intensity and consistency, so too will your appetite. Just focus on the meal in front of you, and remember: you can always drink protein shakes when you can't eat or aren't in the mood to eat. One way or another, though, if you are being active, you need to take in the fuel you require.

The fifth gear is to make food work *for* you, not against you. Consuming a bottle of soda will negatively affect you due to its lack of fiber and its insulin spike, but a bottle of water will hydrate you. Pepperoni pizza will make you feel tired and greasy, whereas fish and rice or trail mix and a piece of fruit will energize you.

The sixth gear is to remain unlimited in your choices. Almost anywhere that you might eat out will offer at least a somewhat healthier option. I recently moved to the South, known for its rich, often fried

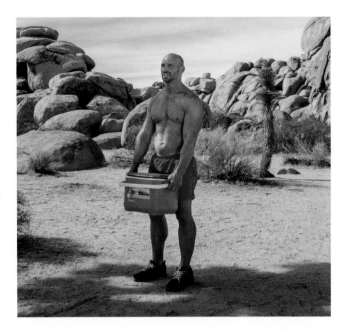

(and delicious) foods. But I needed something quick, cheap, and clean when I was on the go, and I found a chain of fish restaurants that does the trick. Although they have the usual heavy fried fare, there's also grilled tilapia over rice with green beans. Perfect!

LIFE LESSONS

Over the years, my bodyweight has gone up and down. I've had more muscle, less muscle, more body fat, and less body fat. But I've learned that it needn't change much at all. Here are some steps I have implemented to take back control of these fluctuations.

For true nutritional success, aside from what I've already mentioned, you need to change it up. If the idea of one more chicken breast is more than you can bear, switch it up. Do not consume the same foods day in and day out. And use some spices to add interest and flavor to your food.

Humans are not machines. If your body is craving something, give it what it wants. I tend to avoid dairy and juice due to their high sugar content, but sometimes a glass of orange juice or cold whole milk does wonders to reset my body and even my brain. To be human is to be malleable. Eat. Live. Enjoy.

The last lesson is to keep references handy. In my home I have nutrition books, fitness books, fitness clothes, nutritional supplements, and even fitness videos. I keep these items because they help keep me accountable, motivated, passionate, and on the right track. Keep fitness close to your hearts, my friends.

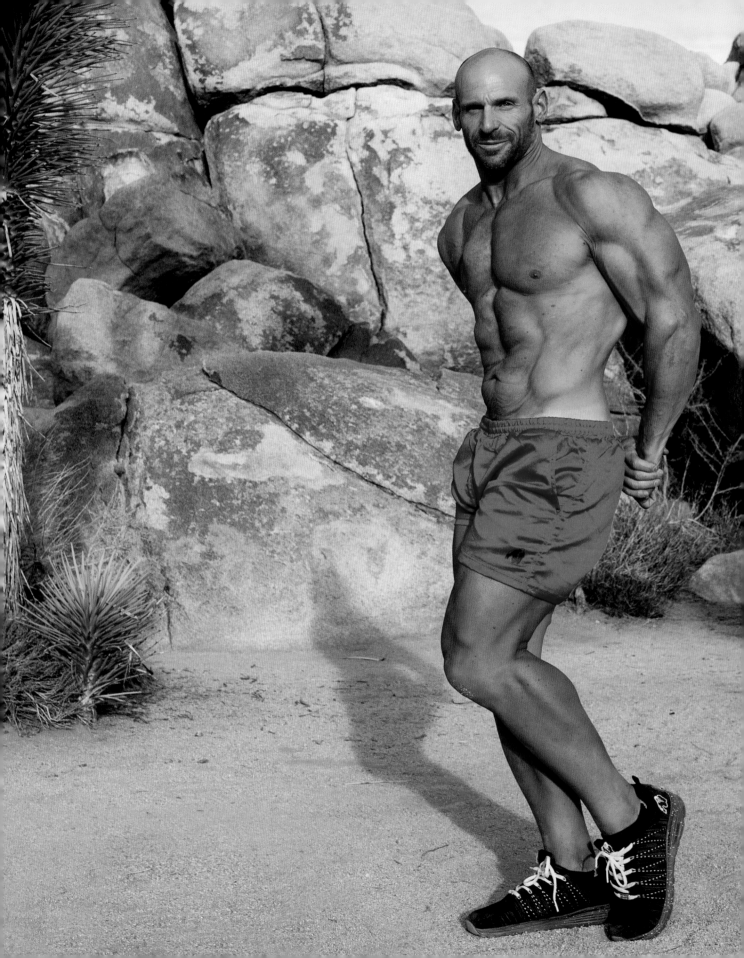

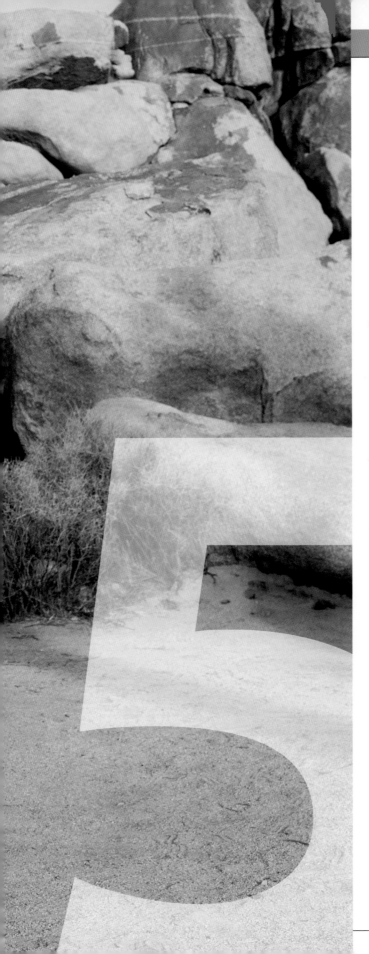

THE
PROGRAM

By understanding and implementing the following key points into your routine, you will achieve more with less. You will take down a tree with fewer, more skilled swings. Since this is a book less about how you look and more about how you function and feel, there are more elements to consider and practice versus the traditional lift, eat, and grow patterns we have previously been exposed to. Breathing, endurance, power, speed, coordination, agility, and flexibility are the pillars of a well-rounded, better, functionally sound you.

Breathing One of the most natural, automatic, and essential of life actions, breathing is often made more complicated than need be. In terms of exercise, inhale or take in air on the lowered, or "negative," portion of an exercise, and exhale on the raised, or "positive," part. On the Elbow Bridge, for example, inhale on the lowering of your body, and exhale upon the raising or completion of the movement. Breathing can also be used to help performance. An explosive exhale on the positive portion can help generate more force during the completion of the repetition.

Endurance A measure of how long your body can exert energy continuously, endurance is not necessarily enhanced through traditional resistance training, with its stop-and-go protocol. But bodyweight exercises in a circuit fashion do help. While training solely for endurance can have a negative impact on strength, the exercises in this book are also designed to enhance your body's natural strength.

Power The amount of force one can exert over time is referred to as power. The faster someone can generate force, the more power they will wield through a given range of motion. Add to this the accuracy applied to a landed movement, and the force will be even more powerful.

Speed While the speed at which you perform exercises should never compromise form or be reliant on momentum (at least for our need here), it can help your workload and repetitions, as long as you know when to use it. By slowing down the negative portion of a repetition, you are effectively loading your muscles for a maximally explosive positive, or finish, portion. Speed should always be coupled with control.

Coordination In short, coordination is the use of several muscles and joints together to complete an action. Good coordination results in smooth, elegant movements.

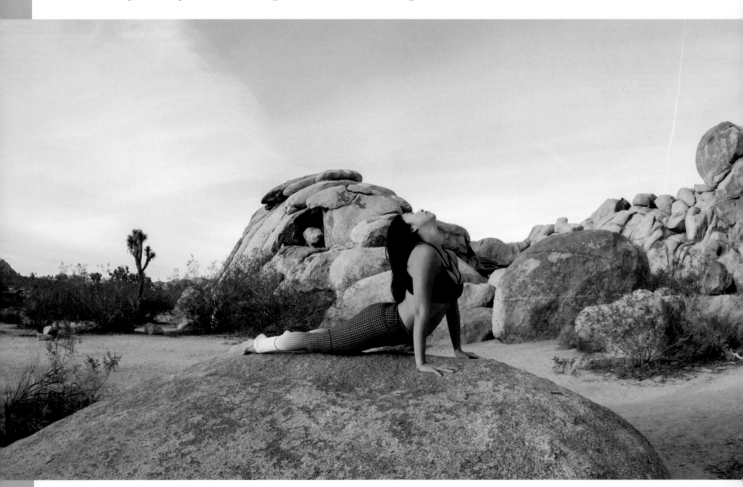

Agility Essential for sportsmen and sportswomen, agility is the ability to change direction or angle of the body efficiently and quickly. The key is, once again, a series of joints and muscles working together to enable movement instantaneously and effectively.

Flexibility The more pliable, or flexible, your muscles are, the greater the range of motion you will have—and therefore the more potential there is for improved performance and muscular composition.

BEHIND THE CROOKED CURTAIN

Just how do these skills work together to improve your fitness? The synergistic combination of bodyweight exercises (utilizing these skills) and good nutrition will bring lean, functional muscle and optimal, long-term results. But why the importance on building muscle? After all, this is not a bodybuilding book.

In terms of true fitness and functional conditioning, lean muscle is still a key aim. Weight gain typically occurs as we age due to less activity and subsequent muscle loss. Our metabolism tends to slow down, and if we continue to eat as we did when we were younger, it will lead to weight gain. By regaining some of that lost muscle, we will renew our metabolism and help slow the accumulation of body fat.

Additionally, cardiovascular work alone is ineffective for muscle building; it simply burns calories that are replaced when we eat our next meal. The need for pure cardio diminishes when many muscles work together repetitively with bodyweight movements. The latter are also superior to isolation exercises, which work well on a specific muscle but do little for groups of muscles acting in unison.

During the course of your workout, you will generally run through a tri-set—three exercises—completing each, resting, and repeating. You then proceed to the next block, as instructed. While each day's workout is different, what they have in common is the thorough working of your body through the three planes of motion for a comprehensive, efficient training regimen.

PERIPHERALS

In terms of additional resistance beyond bodyweight, barbells and the like are not particularly portable. Traditional weightlifting belts, straps, wraps, and so on are no longer necessary for our current physique goals. But a little creativity can go a long way when it comes to enhancing your routine. Sneakers and food coolers,

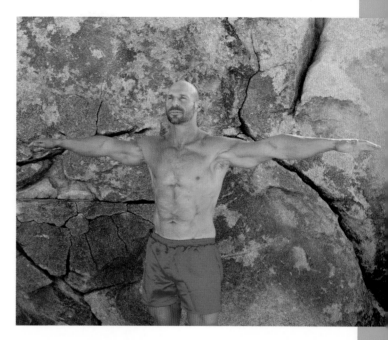

as used in some of the exercises in this book, add variety to an already unique workout. Books can be used as resistance, as can a small dog or even a child. And you can use a regular belt as a rowing exercise tool if you fasten it around an immovable object.

MOVE FREE

We all age; and the older we get, the more issues or excuses we seem to find for putting off training. But the truth is, we have a finite period of personal excellence. This doesn't mean it's all downhill from there, but it does mean things change and may never again be what they once were.

In my early 20s, I suffered a tear to my right pectoralis. It never fully healed, and I never again undertook super-heavy flat bench presses, because this angle places too much tension on the tendons. Instead, I incorporated the incline press into my routine. I refused to let an injury preclude me from an activity I loved. And so should you. Many times in muscle magazines I saw athletes with injuries, a sling around one arm and a pressing movement with the other. These images stayed with me. If world-class athletes can train around an injury, so can the rest of us. As long as it's pain-free. If it hurts, don't do it.

Anytime I have a new client, I always ask if they have any current limitations or injuries. Then, short of them being in a full body cast, I assure them we can work around it. Knee problems? Watch the lunges and

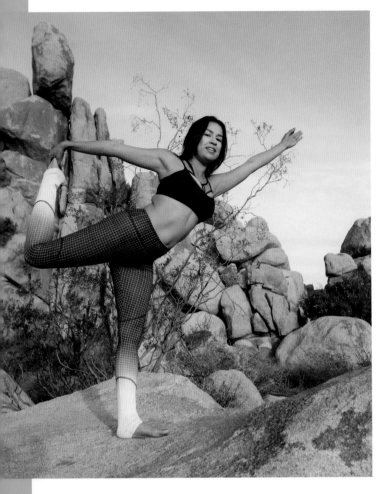

Just as when working out in a gym, the outdoor physique is both built and achieved partially through a series of positions and angles. I've always felt the physique should flow—that is, the eye should travel from muscle group to muscle group upon casual examination and not fixate on one overdeveloped body part at the expense of another.

There should also be effortless lateral, frontal, and transverse movement that is strengthened over time. What good is it to freely press overhead only to be weak or in pain when lifting something from the ground? Here we strive for the smooth paths of motion that we had in our youth.

In the gym, especially with machines, muscles tend to be isolated—a bench press machine works mostly the chest, for example. But a push-up works the chest and ancillary muscles—muscles that must work together to complete a task. The movements and the various angles in this book strengthen groups of muscles to help you get through everyday life.

MOBILITY MOVEMENT

As a young man, I was challenged one day by a braggart who claimed to be faster than me. I couldn't have that (I was young and foolish), so I accepted his challenge. I was quickly in a runner's stance with every muscle tensed and my mind ready. But my body was not. With the go came a quick acceleration and a forced stop. He was long gone, and I was lying on the street in a fetal position. I had no choice but to let him enjoy his win, and I learned a great lesson: Never again would I go from 0 to 100 without a proper warm-up.

When we were children, each gym-class workout was preceded by a warm-up. We were taught that stretching would keep our muscles pliable, increase our range of motion, help prevent injury, and improve performance. Stretching also helps improve muscle recovery, body alignment, and overall posture.

However, on its own, stretching does not improve deficiencies caused by movement or a lack thereof. Neither does it help alleviate pain or dysfunction, or even prevent injury, as previously thought. Stretching alone does little to increase suppleness.

It is only through actual exercise that range of motion is improved. Furthermore, stretching is a rather archaic word that fails to address joint positions. What we are really talking about here is mobilization, which enhances exercise efficiency and improves one's capacity to move.

squats. Shoulder issues? Watch the overhead movements. Neck-fusion surgery? Rest nothing on the neck or rear shoulders. Be cautious, be careful. If it doesn't feel smooth or even mildly good, get out of it, and move onto something else.

I still prefer free weights to machines in these instances, because machines follow a predetermined pathway, whereas weights give you complete freedom. Perhaps even better are bodyweight movements, where not only do you have freedom of movement, but you are also the resistance.

In regards to bodyweight exercises and specifically those found within this book, if it feels off, get out of it, but do remember that you can change the intensity of an exercise simply by shifting its angle. Does a squat feel painful or awkward on your knees? Try moving the legs forward more or spacing your feet differently. You'd be surprised how often this can turn an almost unbearable exercise into a painless yet effective movement.

The mobility movements presented in *Outdoor Physique* can be performed nearly anywhere and will help resolve issues with pain, prevent injury, keep your joints working, and improve your performance. Good movement chiefly comes from two things: joint stability and joint mobility.

Joint stability facilitates the holding or maintaining of joint positions and movements. Stability is the result of nearby tissues working together. Joint mobility refers to how far a joint can move before being restricted by nearby tissue. A lack of stability will have a direct effect on mobility.

The mobility movements presented in this book should be performed prior to exercise. A few minutes on each will prepare your body for the work to follow. Think of it as checking the vitals on the car and then turning the key prior to stepping on the gas.

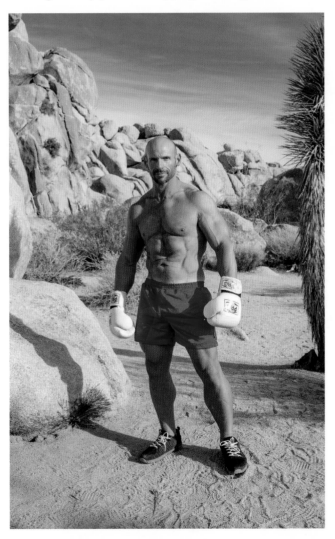

BOXING

Like any complete training program, *Outdoor Physique* includes cardio—but not in the traditional way. In this program you will not cycle endlessly on a stationary bike. You will not slouch over on the StairMaster begging for it to be over. "Okay," you might be thinking, "this is *Outdoor Physique*, so you'll probably have me running sprints and so forth." Nope. Just as sometimes a dog's medicine is placed in peanut butter to disguise it, cardio will find its way into your routine in ways you might not expect. Boxing combinations have been strategically woven in between your circuits to keep your heart rate up, continue burning fat, and increase your stamina and functional conditioning.

Following the bodyweight exercises, you will proceed directly to the boxing portion of your workout, which is done on the honor system, in that there is no counting down from a clock as there is in traditional gym cardio. You simply fire off combinations until you're winded. Start with combination 1 in my list, and work up to combination 6 for Phase 1, then back down, 6 to 1. For Phase 2, combinations 1 to 9 and back; and for Phase 3, combinations 1 to 12 and back. Then repeat. That could take anywhere from 5 minutes to 20 minutes. If you can find a willing partner, you can spice things up by having them call random numbers to you corresponding to specific combinations and blocking your punches with pads.

YOGA

One of the most effective forms of bodyweight exercise, yoga has been included in your journey here in a modified, expedited form. Yoga may be the most ancient type of portable bodyweight training suitable for outdoor use. It improves flexibility, reduces anxiety and stress, increases strength, and helps alleviate pain.

The focus that yoga places on the human body in terms of movement, function, and breathing makes it the perfect counterpart to the other training modalities in this book. And just as Lynn Swann used dance to improve his football performance, you can pair yoga with bodyweight exercises to propel you to new levels of functionality, efficacy, and personal excellence. It will serve as a cool-down after the cardio (boxing) part of your workout. Take your time once locked in a pose, as well as when transitioning to the next pose, remembering to breathe throughout and to remain relaxed.

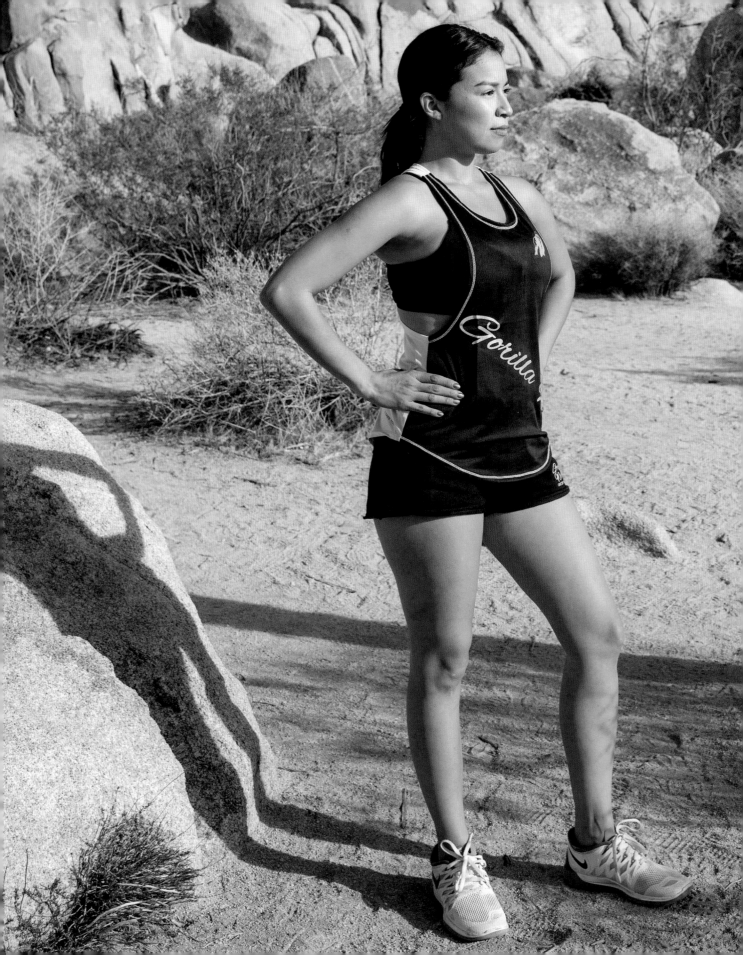

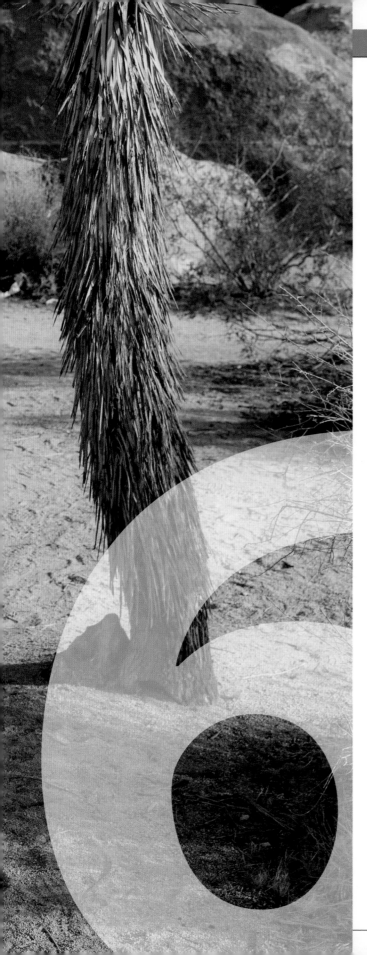

OUTDOOR WORKOUTS

The following plan lists the three phases of the *Outdoor Physique* training protocol, detailing which exercises to perform on each day. Arranged in blocks, the exercises work the body's three planes: sagittal, frontal, and transverse. Complete each exercise and each block as indicated before moving on to the next.

The sequencing of this plan is designed to help keep you motivated and bring the fun back into your workouts. Due to the immediate grouping together of exercises, there is little to no time waiting around between sets. Your muscles work together to perform each movement, and the actions have genuine real-world applications. While you might rarely, if ever, have to perform a bench press in real life, you may well find yourself using the forward motion seen in a Bear Walk.

Outdoor Physique will transform your body for the better, both externally (as we expect of an exercise program) and internally, as you begin to feel and move better. A guy once told me about the money he'd spent in bolting—the process of attaching a house to its concrete foundation—and how, although it will not be seen, it will be important if needed. The same is true of this investment in your body. Have fun!

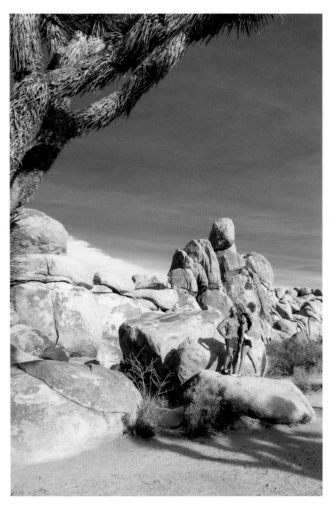

PHASE 1: WEEKS 1–4
BEGINNER TRAINING PROTOCOL

▼ MONDAY

MOBILITY MOVEMENTS
Clam-Shell Stretch, 15 per side
Step and Twist, 15 times per side
Active Hamstring Stretch, 3 times holding for 15-30 seconds per leg
THEN:
Shove-Off, 15-20
Hip-Up, 12-15 per side
Diagonal Mountain Climber, 50
REPEAT THREE TIMES, THEN:
Elbow Bridge, 15-20
Thumbs-Up, 12-15
Squat with Transverse Press, 12-15 per arm
REPEAT THREE TIMES, THEN:
Military Press, 10-15
Side Triceps Extension, 12-15 per side
Diagonal Lunge, 12-15
REPEAT THREE TIMES, THEN:
CARDIO BOXING
Sequence drills: 1-6, 6-1, then repeat.
1. jab
2. jab, cross
3. jab, jab, cross
4. jab, jab, cross, hook
5. jab, jab, cross, hook, duck
6. jab, jab, cross, hook, duck, uppercut
6. jab, jab, cross, hook, duck, uppercut
5. jab, jab, cross, hook, duck
4. jab, jab, cross, hook
3. jab, jab, cross
2. jab, cross
1. jab
BEGINNER YOGA SEQUENCE
Bridge Pose, hold for 8-10 breaths
Child's Pose, hold for 8-10 breaths
Cobra Pose, hold for 8-10 breaths
Downward Dog, hold for 5-8 breaths
Half-Lift, hold for 8-10 breaths
Mountain Pose, hold for 5-8 breaths
Three-Legged Downward Dog, 8-10 breaths, then switch legs
Tree Pose, hold for 8-10 breaths, then switch sides
Warrior 1, hold for 8-10 breaths, then repeat on the other side
Upward Salute, hold for 5-8 breaths

▼ TUESDAY OFF

▼ WEDNESDAY

MOBILITY MOVEMENTS
Clam-Shell Stretch, 15 per side
Step and Twist, 15 times per side
Active Hamstring Stretch, 3 times holding for
    15-30 seconds per leg
THEN:
Bridge Kick, 15-20 per leg
Bent-Over Lateral Raise, 15-20
Hinging Lunge, 12-15 per leg
REPEAT THREE, TIMES, THEN:
Partner Push-Up, 10-15
Side Lunge, 12-15 per leg
Diagonal Crunch with Medicine Ball, 20 per side
REPEAT THREE TIMES, THEN:
Let-Me-Up, 15-20
Squat and Sidekick, 12-15 per leg
Side Plank Rotation, 12-15 per side
REPEAT THREE TIMES, THEN:
CARDIO BOXING
Sequence drills: 1-6, 6-1, then repeat.
1. jab
2. jab, cross
3. jab, jab, cross
4. jab, jab, cross, hook
5. jab, jab, cross, hook, duck
6. jab, jab, cross, hook, duck, uppercut
6. jab, jab, cross, hook, duck, uppercut
5. jab, jab, cross, hook, duck
4. jab, jab, cross, hook
3. jab, jab, cross
2. jab, cross
1. jab
BEGINNER YOGA SEQUENCE
Bridge Pose, hold for 8-10 breaths
Child's Pose, hold for 8-10 breaths
Cobra Pose, hold for 8-10 breaths
Downward Dog, hold for 5-8 breaths
Half-Lift, hold for 8-10 breaths
Mountain Pose, hold for 5-8 breaths
Three-Legged Downward Dog, 8-10 breaths,
    then switch legs
Tree Pose, hold for 8-10 breaths, then switch sides
Warrior 1, hold for 8-10 breaths, then repeat on
    the other side
Upward Salute, hold for 5-8 breaths

▼ THURSDAY OFF

▼ FRIDAY

MOBILITY MOVEMENTS:
Clam-Shell Stretch, 15 per side
Step and Twist, 15 times per side
Active Hamstring Stretch, 3 times holding for 15-30 seconds per leg
THEN:
Handstand with Push-Up, 10-15
Beach Scissors, 15-20 per side
Medicine-Ball Chop, 15-20
REPEAT THREE TIMES, THEN:
Hip Raiser, 15-20
Knee to Shoulder, 20-25 per side
Spider-Man Push-Up, 15-20
REPEAT THREE TIMES, THEN:
Crab Walk, 15-20 steps
Plank Tap, 15-20
Helicopter, 50 per side
REPEAT THREE TIMES, THEN:
CARDIO BOXING
Sequence drills: 1-6, 6-1, then repeat.
1. jab
2. jab, cross
3. jab, jab, cross
4. jab, jab, cross, hook
5. jab, jab, cross, hook, duck
6. jab, jab, cross, hook, duck, uppercut
6. jab, jab, cross, hook, duck, uppercut
5. jab, jab, cross, hook, duck
4. jab, jab, cross, hook
3. jab, jab, cross
2. jab, cross
1. jab
BEGINNER YOGA SEQUENCE
Bridge Pose, hold for 8-10 breaths
Child's Pose, hold for 8-10 breaths
Cobra Pose, hold for 8-10 breaths
Downward Dog, hold for 5-8 breaths
Half-Lift, hold for 8-10 breaths
Mountain Pose, hold for 5-8 breaths
Three-Legged Downward Dog, 8-10 breaths,
    then switch legs
Tree Pose, hold for 8-10 breaths, then switch sides
Warrior 1, hold for 8-10 breaths, then repeat on the other side
Upward Salute, hold for 5-8 breaths

▼ SATURDAY OFF

● SUNDAY OFF

PHASE 2: WEEKS 5–8
INTERMEDIATE TRAINING PROTOCOL

▼ MONDAY

MOBILITY MOVEMENTS
Clam-Shell Stretch, 15 per side
Shoulder Stretch, 3 times, holding for 30 seconds
Step and Twist, 15 times per side
Active Hamstring Stretch, 3 times, holding for 15-30 seconds per leg
THEN:
Seated Dip, 15-20
Lateral Shoulder Raise, 15-20
Russian Twist, 20 per side
REPEAT THREE TIMES, THEN:
Bear Walk, 15-20 steps
Standing Side Leg Lift, 15-20 per leg
Side V-Up, 12-15 per side
REPEAT THREE TIMES, THEN:
Surface Triceps Extension, 15-20
Arm Rotation, 50
Iron Cross, 15 per side
REPEAT THREE TIMES, THEN:
CARDIO BOXING
Sequence drills 1-9, 9-1, then repeat:
1. jab
2. jab, cross
3. jab, jab, cross
4. jab, jab, cross, hook
5. jab, jab, cross, hook, duck
6. jab, jab, cross, hook, duck, uppercut
7. jab, jab, cross, hook, duck, uppercut, jab
8. jab, jab, cross, hook, duck, uppercut, jab, uppercut
9. jab, jab, cross, hook, duck, uppercut, jab, uppercut, duck
9. jab, jab, cross, hook, duck, uppercut, jab, uppercut, duck
8. jab, jab, cross, hook, duck, uppercut, jab, uppercut
7. jab, jab, cross, hook, duck, uppercut, jab
6. jab, jab, cross, hook, duck, uppercut
5. jab, jab, cross, hook, duck
4. jab, jab, cross, hook
3. jab, jab, cross
2. jab, cross
1. jab
INTERMEDIATE YOGA SEQUENCE
Bridge Pose, hold for 8-10 breaths
Child's Pose, hold for 8-10 breaths
Cobra Pose, hold for 8-10 breaths
Downward Dog, hold for 5-8 breaths
Half-Lift, hold for 8-10 breaths

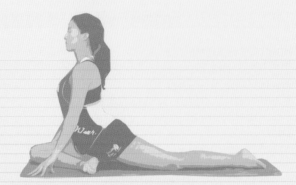

Mountain Pose, hold for 5-8 breaths
Half Lord of the Fishes Pose, 5-8 breaths, then switch sides
Half-Pigeon, hold for 8-10 breaths, then switch sides
Three-Legged Downward Dog, 8-10 breaths, then switch legs
Tree Pose, hold for 8-10 breaths, then switch sides
Warrior 1, hold for 8-10 breaths, then repeat on the other side
Upward Salute, hold for 5-8 breaths
Upward-Facing Dog, hold for 8-10 breaths
Forward Fold, hold for 8-10 breaths

▼ TUESDAY

MOBILITY MOVEMENTS
Clam-Shell Stretch, 15 per side
Shoulder Stretch, 3 times, holding for 30 seconds
Step and Twist, 15 times per side
Active Hamstring Stretch, 3 times, holding for 15-30 seconds per leg
THEN:
Let-Me-In, 15-20
Thumbs-Up, 12-15
Side Plank Rotation, 12-15 per side
REPEAT THREE TIMES, THEN:
Bent-Over Row, 15-20
Squat and Side Kick, 12-15 per side
Side V-Up, 12-15 per side
REPEAT THREE TIMES, THEN:
Single-Leg Bridge, 15-20 per leg
Side Triceps Extension, 12-15 per side
Diagonal Lunge, 12-15 per side
REPEAT THREE TIMES, THEN:
CARDIO BOXING
Sequence drills 1-9, 9-1, then repeat:
1. jab
2. jab, cross
3. jab, jab, cross
4. jab, jab, cross, hook
5. jab, jab, cross, hook, duck
6. jab, jab, cross, hook, duck, uppercut

7. jab, jab, cross, hook, duck, uppercut, jab
8. jab, jab, cross, hook, duck, uppercut, jab, uppercut
9. jab, jab, cross, hook, duck, uppercut, jab, uppercut, duck
9. jab, jab, cross, hook, duck, uppercut, jab, uppercut, duck
8. jab, jab, cross, hook, duck, uppercut, jab, uppercut
7. jab, jab, cross, hook, duck, uppercut, jab
6. jab, jab, cross, hook, duck, uppercut
5. jab, jab, cross, hook, duck
4. jab, jab, cross, hook
3. jab, jab, cross
2. jab, cross
1. jab

INTERMEDIATE YOGA SEQUENCE

Bridge Pose, hold for 8-10 breaths
Child's Pose, hold for 8-10 breaths
Cobra Pose, hold for 8-10 breaths
Downward Dog, hold for 5-8 breaths
Half-Lift, hold for 8-10 breaths
Mountain Pose, hold for 5-8 breaths
Half Lord of the Fishes Pose, 5-8 breaths, then switch sides
Half-Pigeon, hold for 8-10 breaths, then switch sides
Three-Legged Downward Dog, 8-10 breaths, then switch legs
Tree Pose, hold for 8-10 breaths, then switch sides
Warrior 1, hold for 8-10 breaths, then repeat on the other side
Upward Salute, hold for 5-8 breaths
Upward-Facing Dog, hold for 8-10 breaths
Forward Fold, hold for 8-10 breaths

▼ WEDNESDAY OFF

▼ THURSDAY

MOBILITY MOVEMENTS
Clam-Shell Stretch, 15 per side
Shoulder Stretch, 3 times, holding for 30 seconds
Step and Twist, 15 times per side
Active Hamstring Stretch, 3 times, holding for 15-30 seconds per leg
THEN:
Surface Triceps Extension, 15-20
Hip-Up, 12-15 per side
Diagonal Mountain Climber, 50
REPEAT THREE TIMES, THEN:
T-Stand, 15-20 per leg
Beach Scissors, 15-20 per side
Iron Cross, 15 per side
REPEAT THREE TIMES, THEN:
Lower-Back Extension, 15-20
Side Lunge, 12-15 per leg
Spider-Man Push-Up, 15-20

REPEAT THREE TIMES, THEN:
CARDIO BOXING
Sequence drills 1-9, 9-1, then repeat:
1. jab
2. jab, cross
3. jab, jab, cross
4. jab, jab, cross, hook
5. jab, jab, cross, hook, duck
6. jab, jab, cross, hook, duck, uppercut
7. jab, jab, cross, hook, duck, uppercut, jab
8. jab, jab, cross, hook, duck, uppercut, jab, uppercut
9. jab, jab, cross, hook, duck, uppercut, jab, uppercut, duck
9. jab, jab, cross, hook, duck, uppercut, jab, uppercut, duck
8. jab, jab, cross, hook, duck, uppercut, jab, uppercut
7. jab, jab, cross, hook, duck, uppercut, jab
6. jab, jab, cross, hook, duck, uppercut
5. jab, jab, cross, hook, duck
4. jab, jab, cross, hook
3. jab, jab, cross
2. jab, cross
1. jab

INTERMEDIATE YOGA SEQUENCE
Bridge Pose, hold for 8-10 breaths
Child's Pose, hold for 8-10 breaths
Cobra Pose, hold for 8-10 breaths
Downward Dog, hold for 5-8 breaths
Half-Lift, hold for 8-10 breaths
Mountain Pose, hold for 5-8 breaths
Half Lord of the Fishes Pose, 5-8 breaths, then switch sides
Half-Pigeon, hold for 8-10 breaths, then switch sides
Three-Legged Downward Dog, 8-10 breaths,
    then switch legs
Tree Pose, hold for 8-10 breaths, then switch sides
Warrior 1, hold for 8-10 breaths, then repeat on the other side
Upward Salute, hold for 5-8 breaths
Upward-Facing Dog, hold for 8-10 breaths
Forward Fold, hold for 8-10 breaths

▼ FRIDAY

MOBILITY MOVEMENTS
Clam-Shell Stretch, 15 per side
Shoulder Stretch, 3 times, holding for 30 seconds
Step and Twist, 15 times per side
Active Hamstring Stretch, 3 times, holding for 15-30 seconds per leg
THEN:
Ham Sandwich, 12-15
Plank Tap, 15-20
Hinging Lunge, 12-15 per leg

REPEAT THREE TIMES, THEN:
Shrimp Squat, 10-12 per leg
Arm Rotation, 50
Spider-Man Push-Up, 15-20
REPEAT THREE TIMES, THEN:
Double Leg Lift, 20
Knee to Shoulder, 20-25 per side
Diagonal Crunch with Medicine Ball, 20 per side
REPEAT THREE TIMES, THEN:
CARDIO BOXING
Sequence drills 1-9, 9-1, then repeat:
1. jab
2. jab, cross
3. jab, jab, cross
4. jab, jab, cross, hook
5. jab, jab, cross, hook, duck
6. jab, jab, cross, hook, duck, uppercut
7. jab, jab, cross, hook, duck, uppercut, jab
8. jab, jab, cross, hook, duck, uppercut, jab, uppercut
9. jab, jab, cross, hook, duck, uppercut, jab, uppercut, duck
9. jab, jab, cross, hook, duck, uppercut, jab, uppercut, duck
8. jab, jab, cross, hook, duck, uppercut, jab, uppercut
7. jab, jab, cross, hook, duck, uppercut, jab
6. jab, jab, cross, hook, duck, uppercut
5. jab, jab, cross, hook, duck
4. jab, jab, cross, hook
3. jab, jab, cross
2. jab, cross
1. jab
INTERMEDIATE YOGA SEQUENCE
Bridge Pose, hold for 8-10 breaths
Child's Pose, hold for 8-10 breaths
Cobra Pose, hold for 8-10 breaths
Downward Dog, hold for 5-8 breaths
Half-Lift, hold for 8-10 breaths
Mountain Pose, hold for 5-8 breaths
Half Lord of the Fishes Pose, 5-8 breaths, then switch sides
Half-Pigeon, hold for 8-10 breaths, then switch sides
Three-Legged Downward Dog, 8-10 breaths, then switch legs
Tree Pose, hold for 8-10 breaths, then switch sides
Warrior 1, hold for 8-10 breaths, then repeat on the other side
Upward Salute, hold for 5-8 breaths
Upward-Facing Dog, hold for 8-10 breaths
Forward Fold, hold for 8-10 breaths

▼ SATURDAY OFF

● SUNDAY OFF

PHASE 3: WEEKS 9–12 AND BEYOND ADVANCED TRAINING PROTOCOL

▼ MONDAY

MOBILITY MOVEMENTS
Clam-Shell Stretch, 15 per side
Shoulder Stretch, 3 times, holding for 30 seconds
Step and Twist, 15 times per side
Pigeon Pose, 3 times, holding for 30-45 seconds per leg
Active Hamstring Stretch, 3 times, holding for
    15-30 seconds per leg
THEN:
Partner Push-Up, 10-15
Bent-Over Lateral Raises, 15-20
Medicine-Ball Chop, 15-20
Wall Squat, 15-20
REPEAT THREE TIMES, THEN:
Elbow Bridge, 15-20
Lateral Shoulder Raise, 15-20
Squat with Transverse Press, 12-15 per arm
Crab Walk, 15-20 steps
REPEAT THREE TIMES, THEN:
Hip Raiser, 15-20
Standing Side Leg Lift, 15-20 per leg
Russian Twist, 20 per side
Squat, 15-20
REPEAT THREE TIMES, THEN:
CARDIO BOXING
Sequence drills 1-12, 12-1, then repeat:
1. jab
2. jab, cross
3. jab, jab, cross
4. jab, jab, cross, hook
5. jab, jab, cross, hook, duck
6. jab, jab, cross, hook, duck, uppercut
7. jab, jab, cross, hook, duck, uppercut, jab
8. jab, jab, cross, hook, duck, uppercut, jab, uppercut
9. jab, jab, cross, hook, duck, uppercut, jab, uppercut, duck
10. jab, jab, cross, hook, duck, uppercut, jab, uppercut, duck, jab
11. jab, jab, cross, hook, duck, uppercut, jab, uppercut, duck, jab, cross
12. jab, jab, cross, hook, duck, uppercut, jab, uppercut, duck, jab, cross, jab
12. jab, jab, cross, hook, duck, uppercut, jab, uppercut, duck, jab, cross, jab
11. jab, jab, cross, hook, duck, uppercut, jab, uppercut, duck, jab, cross
10. jab, jab, cross, hook, duck, uppercut, jab, uppercut, duck, jab
9. jab, jab, cross, hook, duck, uppercut, jab, uppercut, duck
8. jab, jab, cross, hook, duck, uppercut, jab, uppercut
7. jab, jab, cross, hook, duck, uppercut, jab
6. jab, jab, cross, hook, duck, uppercut

5. jab, jab, cross, hook, duck
4. jab, jab, cross, hook
3. jab, jab, cross
2. jab, cross
1. jab

ADVANCED YOGA SEQUENCE

Bridge Pose, hold for 8-10 breaths
Child's Pose, hold for 8-10 breaths
Cobra Pose, hold for 8-10 breaths
Downward Dog, hold for 5-8 breaths
Half-Lift, hold for 8-10 breaths
Mountain Pose, hold for 5-8 breaths
One-Legged Bridge Pointing Upward, hold for 8-10 seconds, lower, and repeat with the other leg
Half Lord of the Fishes Pose, 5-8 breaths, then switch sides
Half Pigeon, hold for 8-10 breaths, then switch sides
Three-Legged Downward Dog, 8-10 breaths, then switch legs
Tree Pose, hold for 8-10 breaths, then switch sides
Triangle Pose, 5-8 breaths, then switch sides
Warrior 1, hold for 8-10 breaths, then repeat on the other side
Upward Salute, hold for 5-8 breaths
Upward-Facing Dog, hold for 8-10 breaths
Warrior 3, hold for 8-10 breaths, then switch sides
Forward Fold, hold for 8-10 breaths

▼ TUESDAY

MOBILITY MOVEMENTS

Clam-Shell Stretch, 15 per side
Shoulder Stretch, 3 times, holding for 30 seconds
Step and Twist, 15 times per side
Pigeon Pose, 3 times, holding for 30-45 per leg
Active Hamstring Stretch, 3 times, holding for 15-30 seconds per leg

THEN:

Shove-Off, 15-20
Plank Tap, 15-20
Helicopter, 50
Military Press, 10-15

REPEAT THREE TIMES, THEN:

Let-Me-In, 15-20
Thumbs-Up, 12-15
Side V-Up, 12-15 per side
T-Stand, 15-20 per leg

REPEAT THREE TIMES, THEN:

Let-Me-Up, 15-20
Side Triceps Extension, 12-15 per side
Diagonal Lunge, 12-15 per side
Butt Kick, 50 per leg

REPEAT THREE TIMES, THEN:
CARDIO BOXING

Sequence drills 1–12, 12–1, then repeat:
1. jab
2. jab, cross
3. jab, jab, cross
4. jab, jab, cross, hook
5. jab, jab, cross, hook, duck
6. jab, jab, cross, hook, duck, uppercut
7. jab, jab, cross, hook, duck, uppercut, jab
8. jab, jab, cross, hook, duck, uppercut, jab, uppercut
9. jab, jab, cross, hook, duck, uppercut, jab, uppercut, duck
10. jab, jab, cross, hook, duck, uppercut, jab, uppercut, duck, jab
11. jab, jab, cross, hook, duck, uppercut, jab, uppercut, duck, jab, cross
12. jab, jab, cross, hook, duck, uppercut, jab, uppercut, duck, jab, cross, jab
12. jab, jab, cross, hook, duck, uppercut, jab, uppercut, duck, jab, cross, jab
11. jab, jab, cross, hook, duck, uppercut, jab, uppercut, duck, jab, cross
10. jab, jab, cross, hook, duck, uppercut, jab, uppercut, duck, jab
9. jab, jab, cross, hook, duck, uppercut, jab, uppercut, duck
8. jab, jab, cross, hook, duck, uppercut, jab, uppercut
7. jab, jab, cross, hook, duck, uppercut, jab
6. jab, jab, cross, hook, duck, uppercut
5. jab, jab, cross, hook, duck
4. jab, jab, cross, hook
3. jab, jab, cross
2. jab, cross
1. jab

ADVANCED YOGA SEQUENCE

Bridge Pose, hold for 8-10 breaths
Child's Pose, hold for 8-10 breaths
Cobra Pose, hold for 8-10 breaths
Downward Dog, hold for 5-8 breaths
Half-Lift, hold for 8-10 breaths
Mountain Pose, hold for 5-8 breaths
One-Legged Bridge Pointing Upward, hold for 8-10 seconds, lower, and repeat with the other leg
Half Lord of the Fishes Pose, 5-8 breaths, then switch sides
Half-Pigeon, hold for 8-10 breaths, then switch sides
Three-Legged Downward Dog, 8-10 breaths, then switch legs
Tree Pose, hold for 8-10 breaths, then switch sides
Triangle Pose, 5-8 breaths, then switch sides
Warrior 1, hold for 8-10 breaths, then repeat on the other side
Upward Salute, hold for 5-8 breaths
Upward-Facing Dog, hold for 8-10 breaths
Warrior 3, hold for 8-10 breaths, then switch sides
Forward Fold, hold for 8-10 breaths

▼ WEDNESDAY OFF

▼ THURSDAY

MOBILITY MOVEMENTS
Clam Shell Stretch, 15 per side
Shoulder Stretch, 3 times, holding for 30 seconds
Step and Twist, 15 times per side
Pigeon Pose, 3 times, holding for 30-45 seconds per leg
Active Hamstring Stretch, 3 times, holding for 15-30 seconds per leg

THEN:
Bridge Kick, 15-20 per leg
Knee to Shoulder, 20-25 per side
Side-Plank Rotation, 12-15 per side
Seated Dip, 15-20

REPEAT THREE TIMES, THEN:
Handstand with Push-Up, 10-15
Hip-Up, 12-15 per side
Helicopter, 50 per side
Squat, 15-20

REPEAT THREE TIMES, THEN:
Bear Walk, 15-20 steps
Lateral Shoulder Raise, 15-20
Hinging Lunge, 12-15 per leg
Medicine-Ball Sit-Up, 20

REPEAT THREE TIMES, THEN:

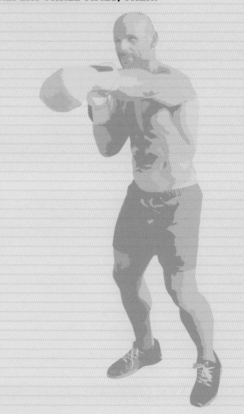

CARDIO BOXING
Sequence drills 1-12, 12-1, then repeat:
1. jab
2. jab, cross
3. jab, jab, cross
4. jab, jab, cross, hook
5. jab, jab, cross, hook, duck
6. jab, jab, cross, hook, duck, uppercut
7. jab, jab, cross, hook, duck, uppercut, jab
8. jab, jab, cross, hook, duck, uppercut, jab, uppercut
9. jab, jab, cross, hook, duck, uppercut, jab, uppercut, duck
10. jab, jab, cross, hook, duck, uppercut, jab, uppercut, duck, jab
11. jab, jab, cross, hook, duck, uppercut, jab, uppercut, duck, jab, cross
12. jab, jab, cross, hook, duck, uppercut, jab, uppercut, duck, jab, cross, jab
12. jab, jab, cross, hook, duck, uppercut, jab, uppercut, duck, jab, cross, jab
11. jab, jab, cross, hook, duck, uppercut, jab, uppercut, duck, jab, cross
10. jab, jab, cross, hook, duck, uppercut, jab, uppercut, duck, jab
9. jab, jab, cross, hook, duck, uppercut, jab, uppercut, duck
8. jab, jab, cross, hook, duck, uppercut, jab, uppercut
7. jab, jab, cross, hook, duck, uppercut, jab
6. jab, jab, cross, hook, duck, uppercut
5. jab, jab, cross, hook, duck
4. jab, jab, cross, hook
3. jab, jab, cross
2. jab, cross
1. jab

ADVANCED YOGA SEQUENCE
Bridge Pose, hold for 8-10 breaths
Child's Pose, hold for 8-10 breaths
Cobra Pose, hold for 8-10 breaths
Downward Dog, hold for 5-8 breaths
Half-Lift, hold for 8-10 breaths
Mountain Pose, hold for 5-8 breaths
One-Legged Bridge Pointing Upward, hold for 8-10 seconds, lower, and repeat with the other leg
Half Lord of the Fishes Pose, 5-8 breaths, then switch sides
Half-Pigeon, hold for 8-10 breaths, then switch sides
Three-Legged Downward Dog, 8-10 breaths, then switch legs
Tree Pose, hold for 8-10 breaths, then switch sides
Triangle Pose, 5-8 breaths, then switch sides
Warrior 1, hold for 8-10 breaths, then repeat on the other side
Upward Salute, hold for 5-8 breaths
Upward-Facing Dog, hold for 8-10 breaths
Warrior 3, hold for 8-10 breaths, then switch sides
Forward Fold, hold for 8-10 breaths

▼ FRIDAY

MOBILITY MOVEMENTS

Clam-Shell Stretch, 15 per side
Shoulder Stretch, 3 times, holding for 30 seconds
Step and Twist, 15 times per side
Pigeon Pose, 3 times, holding for 30-45 seconds per leg
Active Hamstring Stretch, 3 times, holding for 15-30 seconds per leg

THEN:

Bent-Over Row, 15-20
Squat and Sidekick, 12-15 per leg
Diagonal Crunch with Medicine Ball, 20 per side
Standing Calf Raise, 15-20

REPEAT THREE TIMES, THEN:

Lower-Back Extension, 15-20
Bent-Over Lateral Raise, 15-20
Squat with Transverse Press, 12-15 per arm
Ham Sandwich, 12-15

REPEAT THREE TIMES, THEN:

Shrimp Squat, 10-12 per leg
Beach Scissors, 15-20 per side
Russian Twist, 20 per side
Double Leg Lift, 20

REPEAT THREE TIMES, THEN:

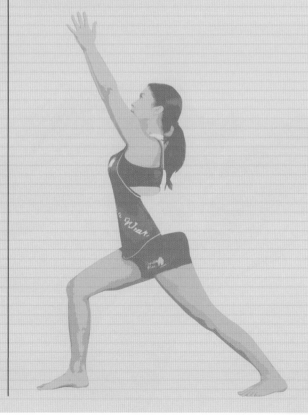

CARDIO BOXING

Sequence drills 1-12, 12-1, then repeat:
1. jab
2. jab, cross
3. jab, jab, cross
4. jab, jab, cross, hook
5. jab, jab, cross, hook, duck
6. jab, jab, cross, hook, duck, uppercut
7. jab, jab, cross, hook, duck, uppercut, jab
8. jab, jab, cross, hook, duck, uppercut, jab, uppercut
9. jab, jab, cross, hook, duck, uppercut, jab, uppercut, duck
10. jab, jab, cross, hook, duck, uppercut, jab, uppercut, duck, jab
11. jab, jab, cross, hook, duck, uppercut, jab, uppercut, duck, jab, cross
12. jab, jab, cross, hook, duck, uppercut, jab, uppercut, duck, jab, cross, jab
12. jab, jab, cross, hook, duck, uppercut, jab, uppercut, duck, jab, cross, jab
11. jab, jab, cross, hook, duck, uppercut, jab, uppercut, duck, jab, cross
10. jab, jab, cross, hook, duck, uppercut, jab, uppercut, duck, jab
9. jab, jab, cross, hook, duck, uppercut, jab, uppercut, duck
8. jab, jab, cross, hook, duck, uppercut, jab, uppercut
7. jab, jab, cross, hook, duck, uppercut, jab
6. jab, jab, cross, hook, duck, uppercut
5. jab, jab, cross, hook, duck
4. jab, jab, cross, hook
3. jab, jab, cross
2. jab, cross
1. jab

ADVANCED YOGA SEQUENCE

Bridge Pose, hold for 8-10 breaths
Child's Pose, hold for 8-10 breaths
Cobra Pose, hold for 8-10 breaths
Downward Dog, hold for 5-8 breaths
Half-Lift, hold for 8-10 breaths
Mountain Pose, hold for 5-8 breaths
One-Legged Bridge Pointing Upward, hold for 8-10 seconds, lower, and repeat with the other leg
Half Lord of the Fishes Pose, 5-8 breaths, then switch sides
Half-Pigeon, hold for 8-10 breaths, then switch sides
Three-Legged Downward Dog, 8-10 breaths, then switch legs
Tree Pose, hold for 8-10 breaths, then switch sides
Triangle Pose, 5-8 breaths, then switch sides
Warrior 1, hold for 8-10 breaths, then repeat on the other side
Upward Salute, hold for 5-8 breaths
Upward-Facing Dog, hold for 8-10 breaths
Warrior 3, hold for 8-10 breaths, then switch sides
Forward Fold, hold for 8-10 breaths

▼ SATURDAY OFF

● SUNDAY OFF

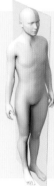

THE SAGITTAL PLANE runs through the center of the body, dividing it into left and right halves. Forward and backward movements along this plane are called sagittal.

PRIMARY MUSCLE ACTION

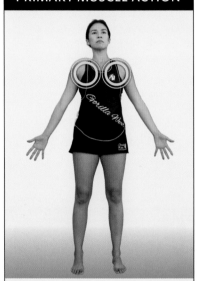

- Pectorals
- Shoulders
- Triceps

SHOVE-OFF

PROGRESSION

1 Stand before a stable angled surface with your arms extended.

2 In a controlled manner, fall forward until your palms are touching the surface, and lower yourself until your chest is nearly touching the surface.

3 Explosively push yourself off the surface until you are standing, and complete 15–20 repetitions.

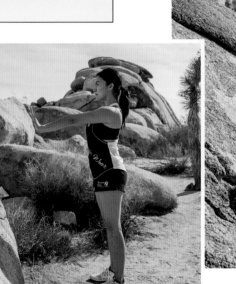

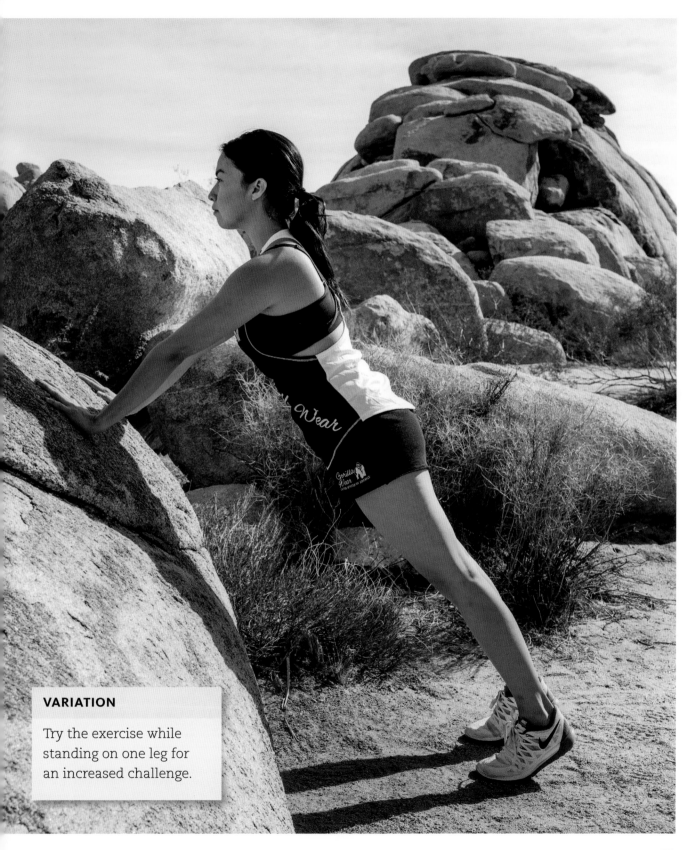

VARIATION

Try the exercise while standing on one leg for an increased challenge.

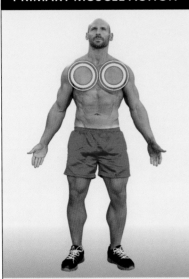

- Pectorals
- Deltoids
- Triceps

PARTNER PUSH-UP

PROGRESSION

1 Lie face down in a traditional push-up position.

2 Have your partner lie along your body, facing upward with their arms crossed.

3 Push up to full extension, lower, and complete 10–15 repetitions.

VARIATION

Try the exercise with one leg raised out to the side for an increased challenge.

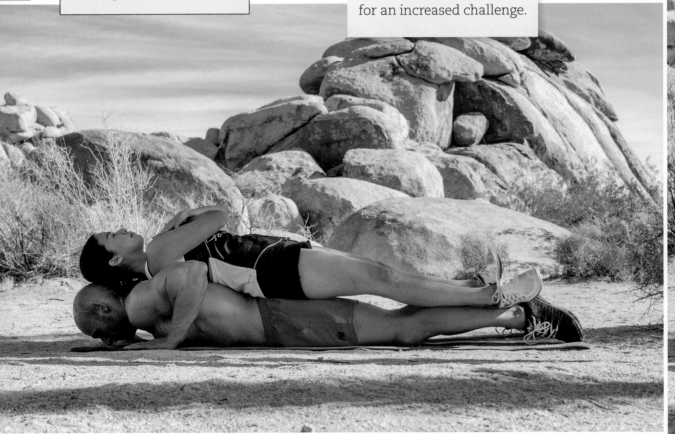

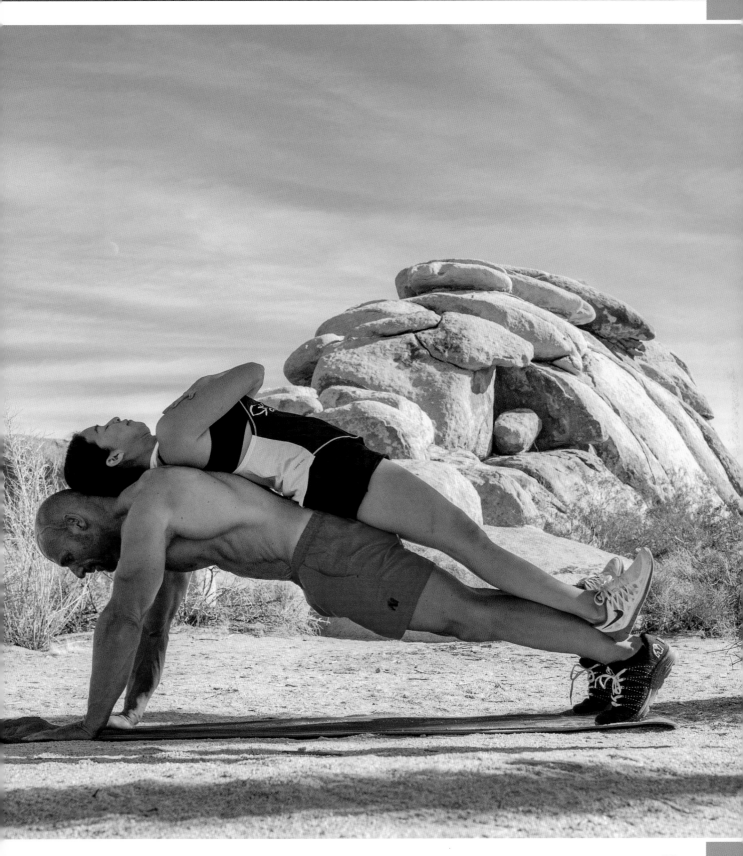

PRIMARY MUSCLE ACTION

- Upper Back
- Triceps
- Core

ELBOW BRIDGE

PROGRESSION

1 Lie on your back with your arms bent at a 90-degree angle at your sides, fists skyward, and your legs bent and shoulder-width apart.

2 Push through your elbows and triceps as you raise your pelvis until your body is largely in a straight line.

3 Lower in a controlled manner, and complete 15–20 repetitions.

VARIATION

Try this exercise with one leg raised for an increased challenge.

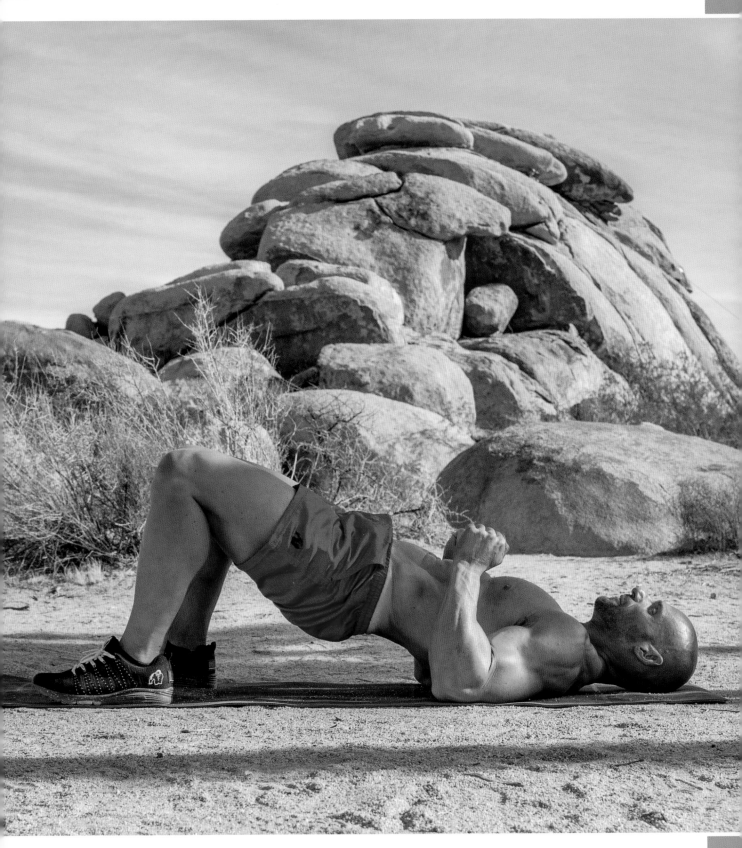

PRIMARY MUSCLE ACTION

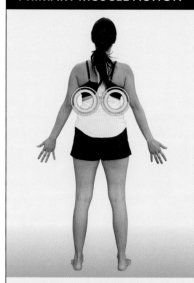

- Lats
- Posterior Deltoids
- Biceps and Forearms

LET-ME-IN

PROGRESSION

1 Facing a steady structure, grab both sides with your hands while digging your heels into the ground for stabilization.

2 Lean back while keeping your arms straight, your back flat, and your rear out as you bend at the knees until your thighs are parallel to the ground.

3 Pull yourself back up and inward, until your chest is close to the structure, and complete 15–20 repetitions.

VARIATION

Try this exercise with one foot raised for an increased challenge.

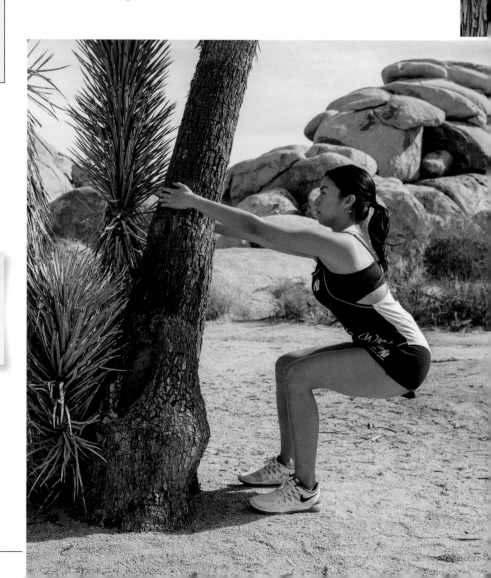

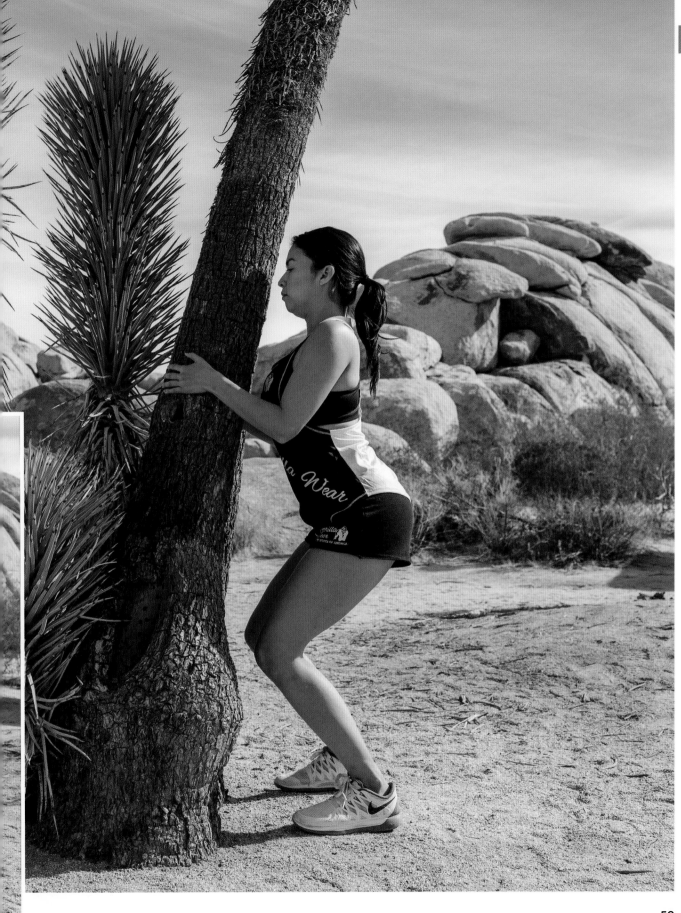

PRIMARY MUSCLE ACTION

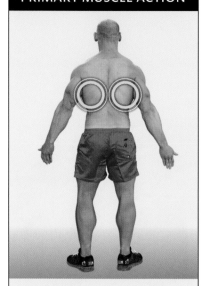

- Lats
- Posterior Deltoids
- Biceps and Forearms

LET-ME-UP

PROGRESSION

1 Lie back beneath a sturdy overhead object, holding with both hands and bending your legs.

2 Line up your chest directly beneath said object, and pull yourself upward until your chest is nearly touching it.

3 Lower to arms' length, and complete 15–20 repetitions.

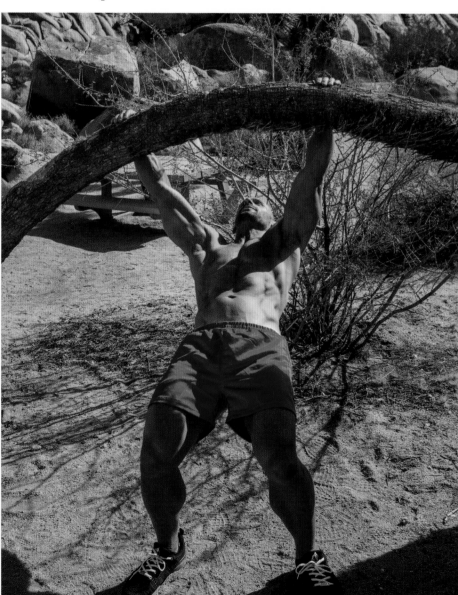

VARIATION

Try this exercise with one foot raised for an increased challenge.

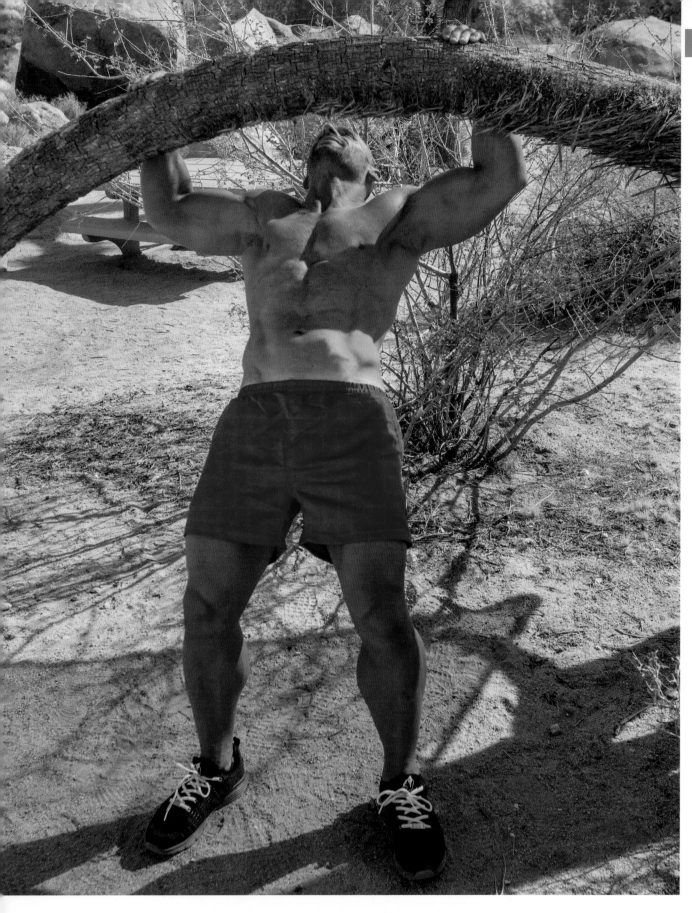

PRIMARY MUSCLE ACTION

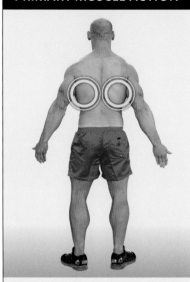

- Lats
- Core

BENT-OVER ROW

PROGRESSION

1 In a standing position, holding a cooler or other portable object as resistance, bend forward at the waist while maintaining a flat back with legs slightly bent.

2 Allowing your arms to dangle directly below you, pull the object into your lower abdomen.

3 Squeeze your shoulder blades together, lower, and complete 15–20 repetitions.

VARIATION

Try this exercise while standing on one leg for an increased challenge.

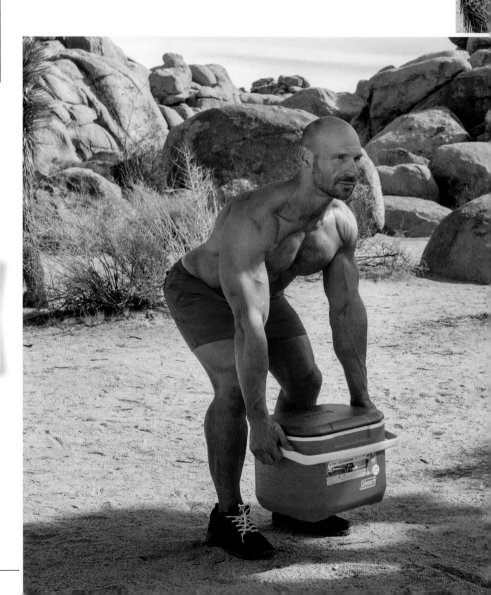

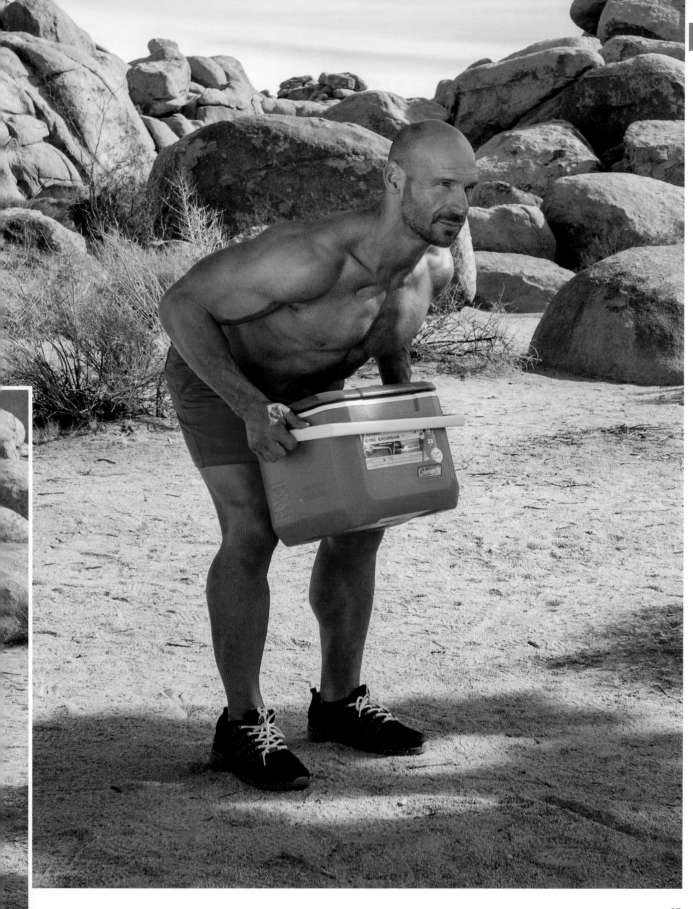

LOWER-BACK EXTENSION

PROGRESSION

PRIMARY MUSCLE ACTION

- Spinal Erectors

1 Lie face down on a mat, with your hands clasped behind your head and your feet close together.

2 Raise upward from your torso until you feel a contraction in your lower back.

3 Lower, and complete 15–20 repetitions.

VARIATION

Try this exercise with your arms outstretched in front and your legs spaced wider apart.

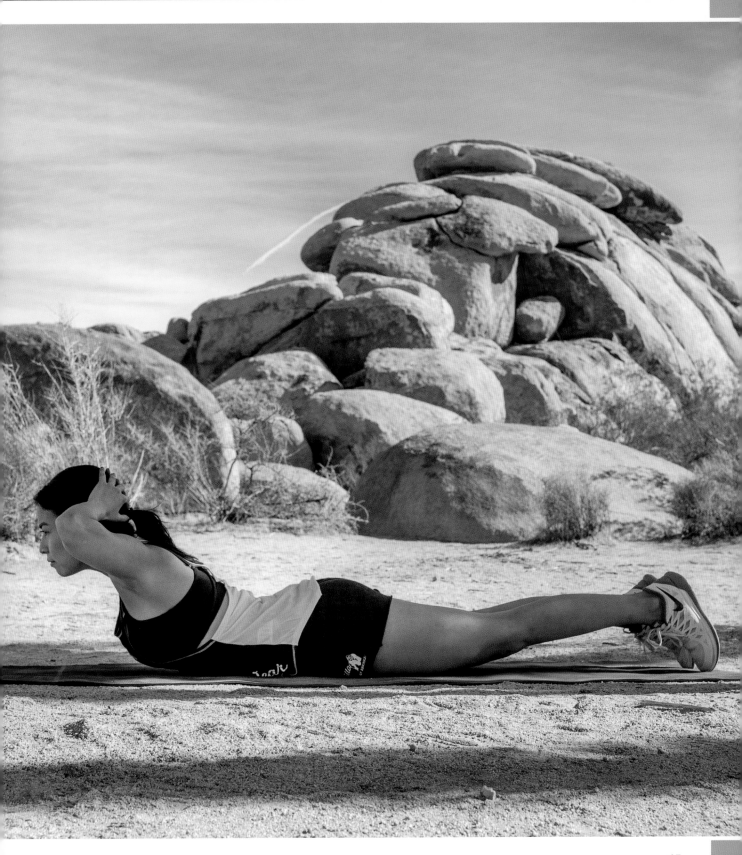

PRIMARY MUSCLE ACTION

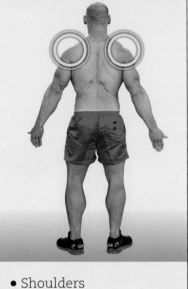

- Shoulders
- Pectorals
- Triceps
- Trapezius
- Core

BEAR WALK

PROGRESSION

1 Place your hands and toes on the ground a few feet from one another.

2 Crawl forward while keeping close to the ground for 15–20 steps.

VARIATION

Try crawling backward for an increased challenge.

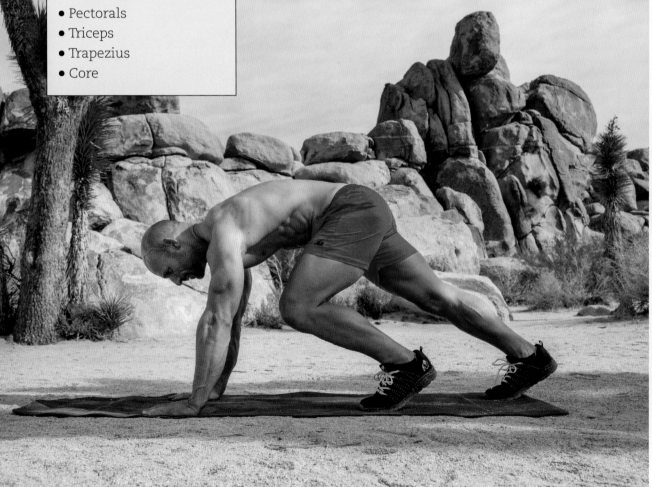

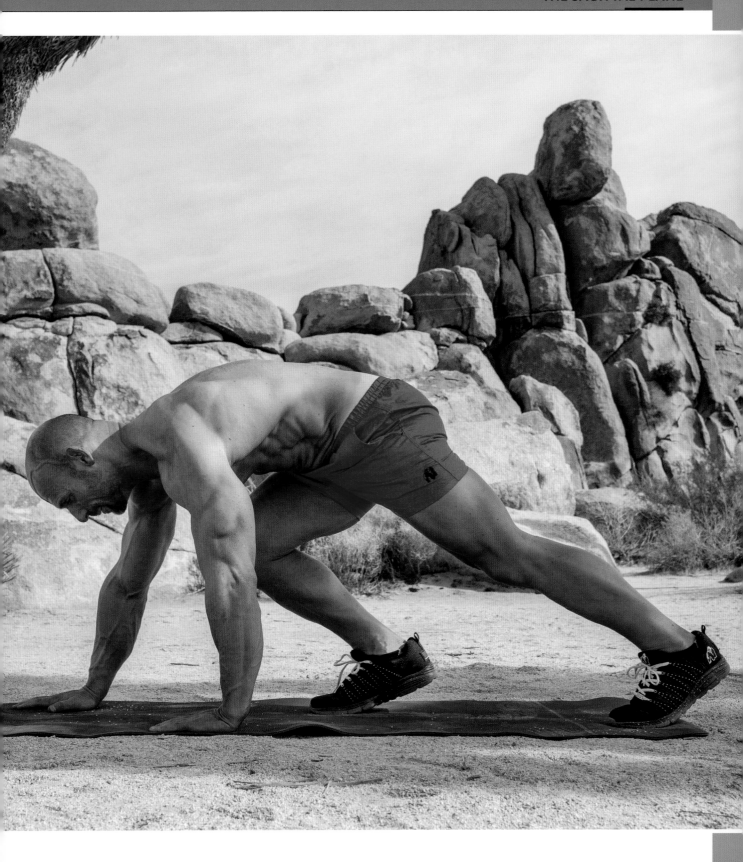

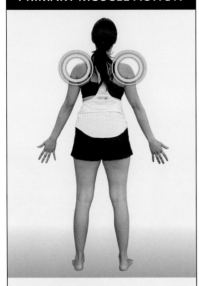

- Shoulders
- Triceps

MILITARY PRESS

PROGRESSION

1 Stand with your heels close together, then bend forward and plant your hands in front at arms' length.

2 Maintain a straight back while thrusting your rear in the air, keeping your head between your hands.

3 Bend your arms and lower your torso until your head is near the ground.

4 Push back up to full arm extension, and complete 10–15 repetitions.

VARIATION

Try this exercise with one leg raised behind you for an increased challenge.

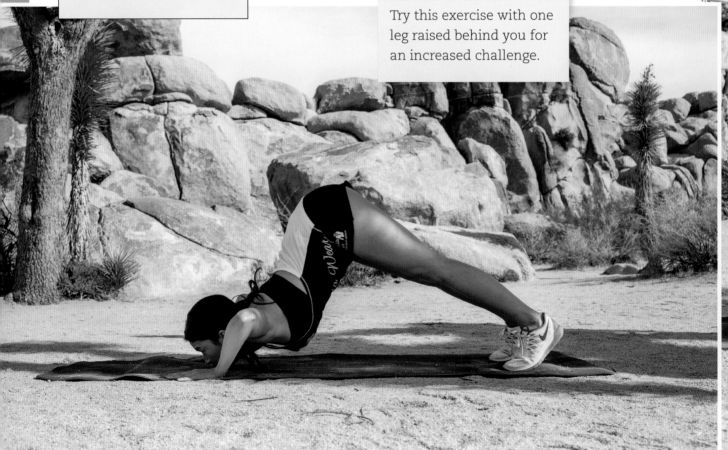

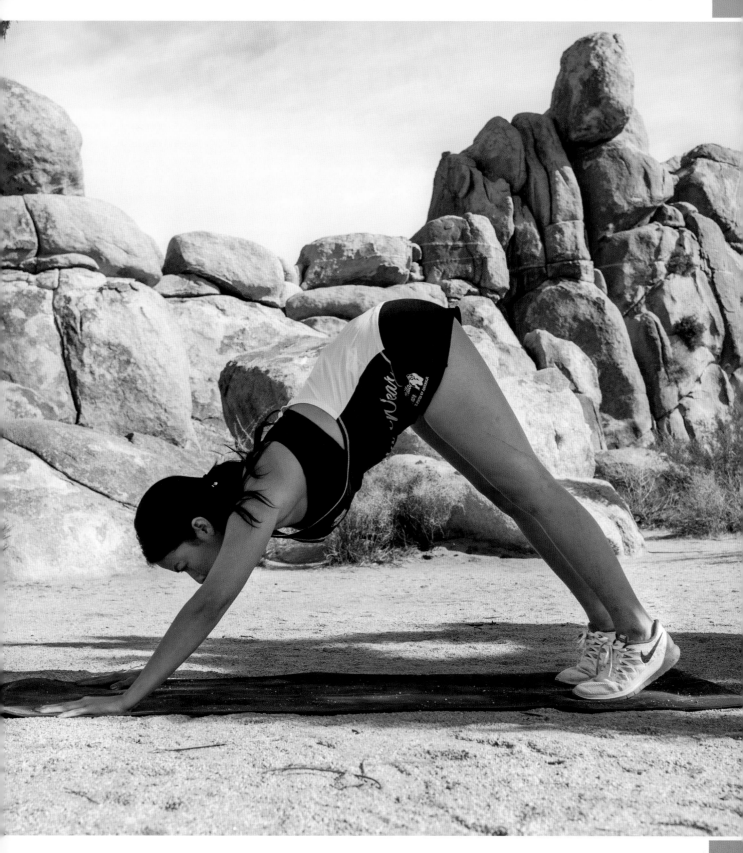

HANDSTAND WITH PUSH-UP

PRIMARY MUSCLE ACTION

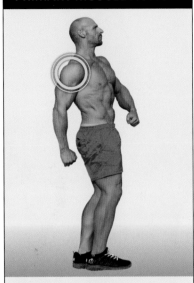

- Deltoids
- Triceps
- Core

PROGRESSION

1 Plant your hands on the ground while facing a vertical sturdy object, then hoist your legs up against the surface until your body is one straight upside-down line.

2 Bend your arms and slowly lower your head toward the ground, without touching it.

3 Push back up to full arm extension, and complete 10–15 repetitions.

VARIATION

Make this exercise easier by having a partner hold your legs.

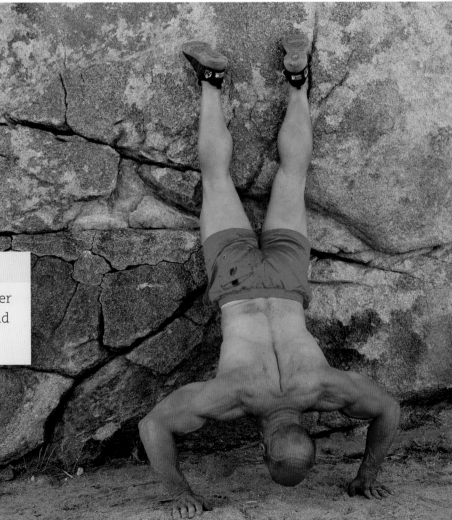

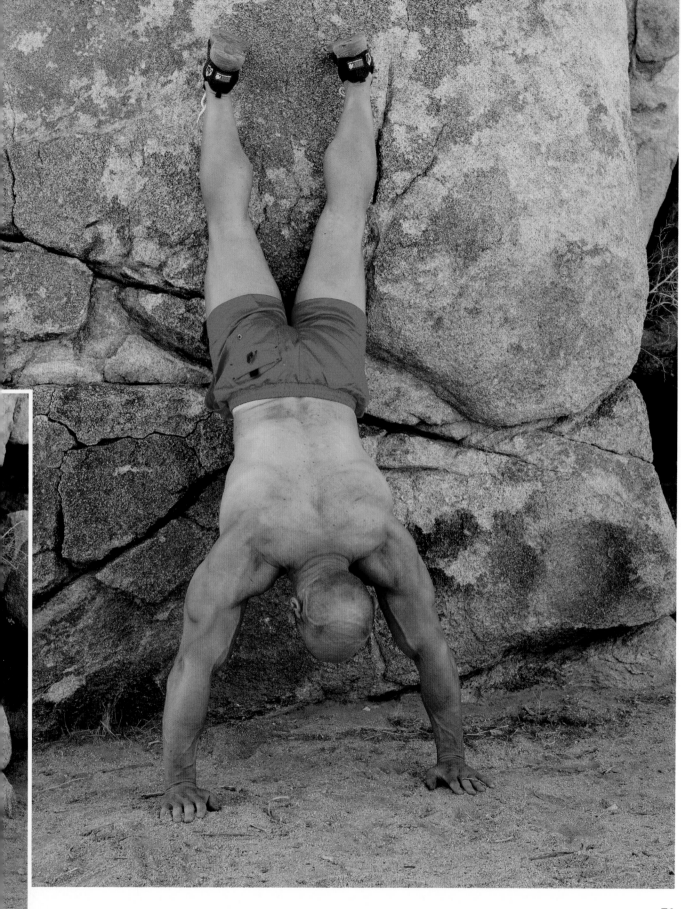

BRIDGE KICK

PRIMARY MUSCLE ACTION

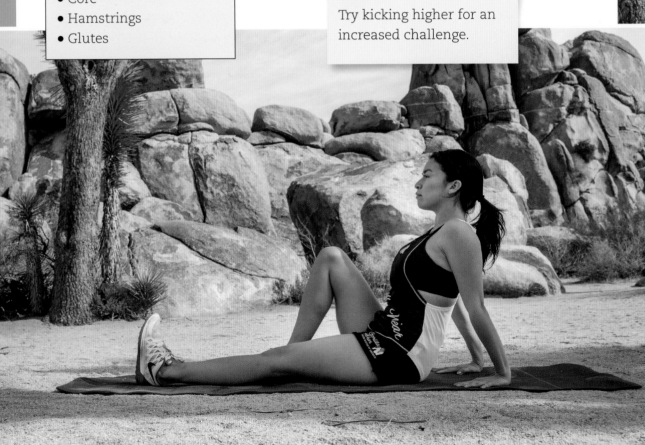

- Triceps
- Core
- Hamstrings
- Glutes

PROGRESSION

1 Begin seated with one leg in front of you and the other bent, your arms behind you, and your palms facing forward while you lean back slightly.

2 Push through your palms while you raise your pelvis, extending the straight leg upward.

3 Lower, complete 15–20 repetitions, then switch legs.

VARIATION

Try kicking higher for an increased challenge.

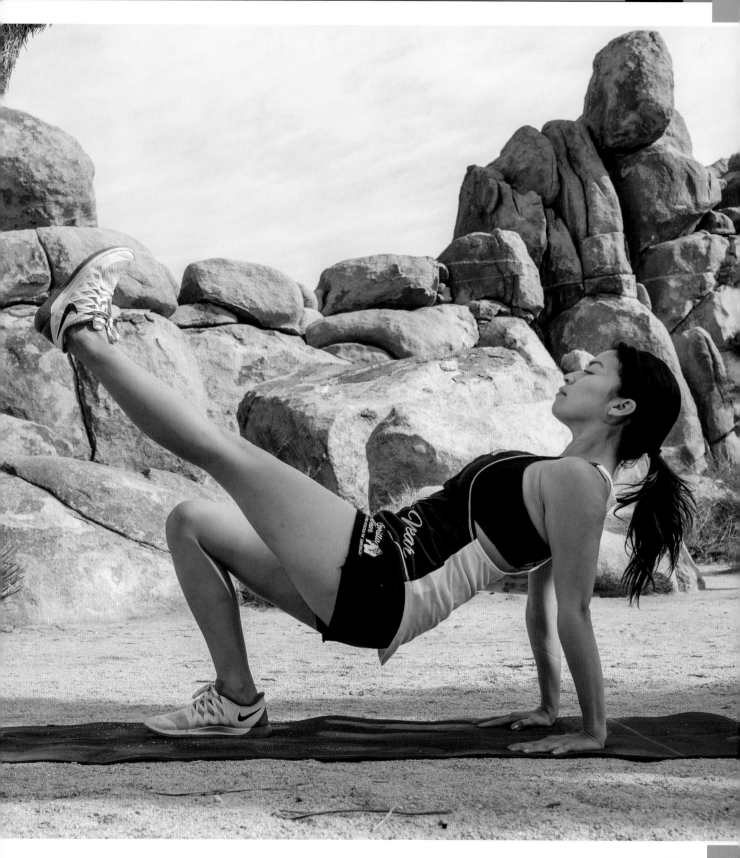

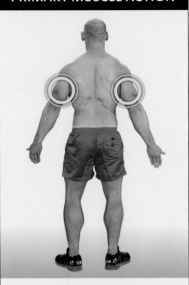

PRIMARY MUSCLE ACTION

• Triceps

SEATED DIP

PROGRESSION

1 With your rear braced against a stable surface, such as a picnic bench set, place your hands near your hips and stretch your legs in front of you with your toes facing upward.

2 Lower yourself while bending your arms at the elbow until at roughly a 90-degree angle.

3 Push yourself back up until your arms are straight, and complete 15–20 repetitions.

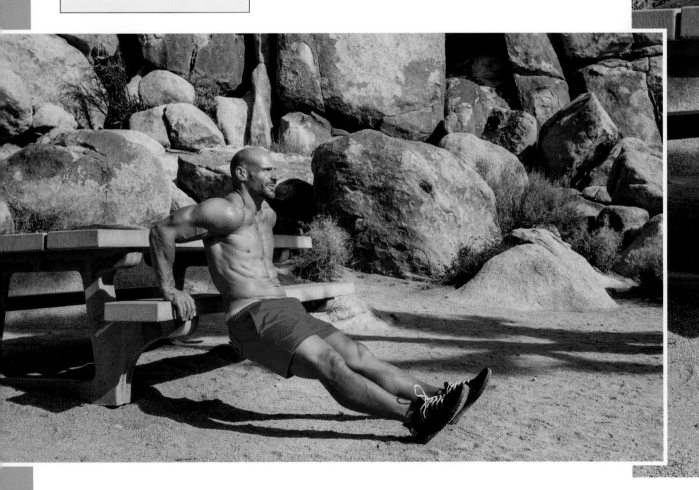

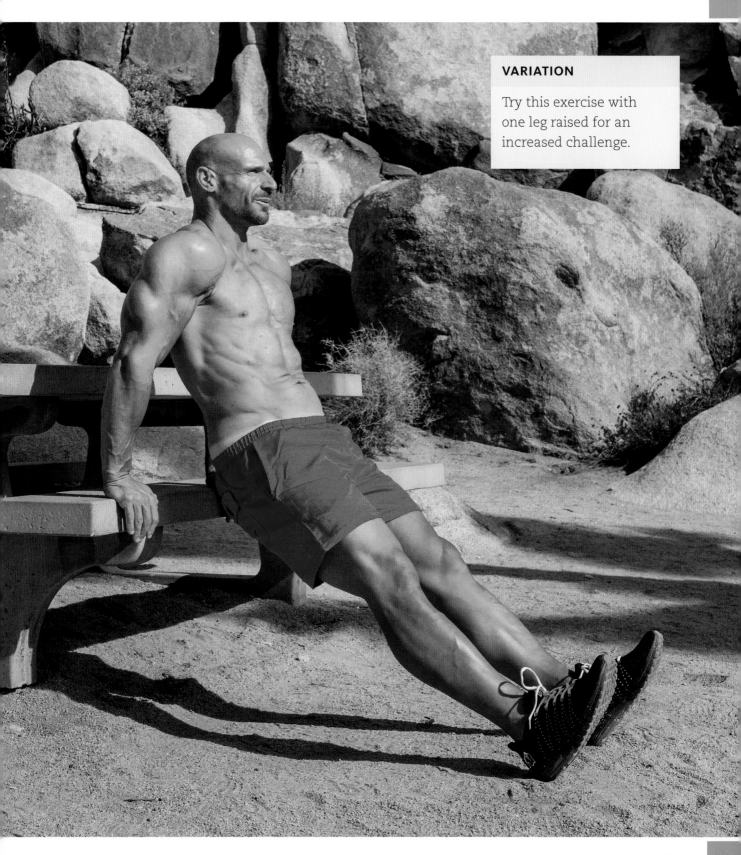

VARIATION

Try this exercise with
one leg raised for an
increased challenge.

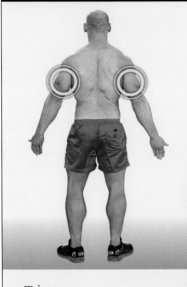

PRIMARY MUSCLE ACTION

- Triceps

CRAB WALK

PROGRESSION

1 In a seated position with bent legs, place your hands at your sides, palms down and facing forward.

2 Raise your glutes off the ground, and walk forward for 15–20 steps.

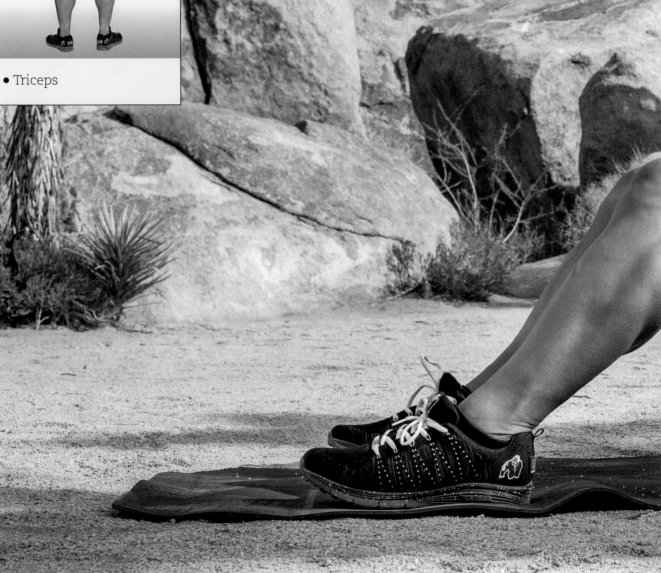

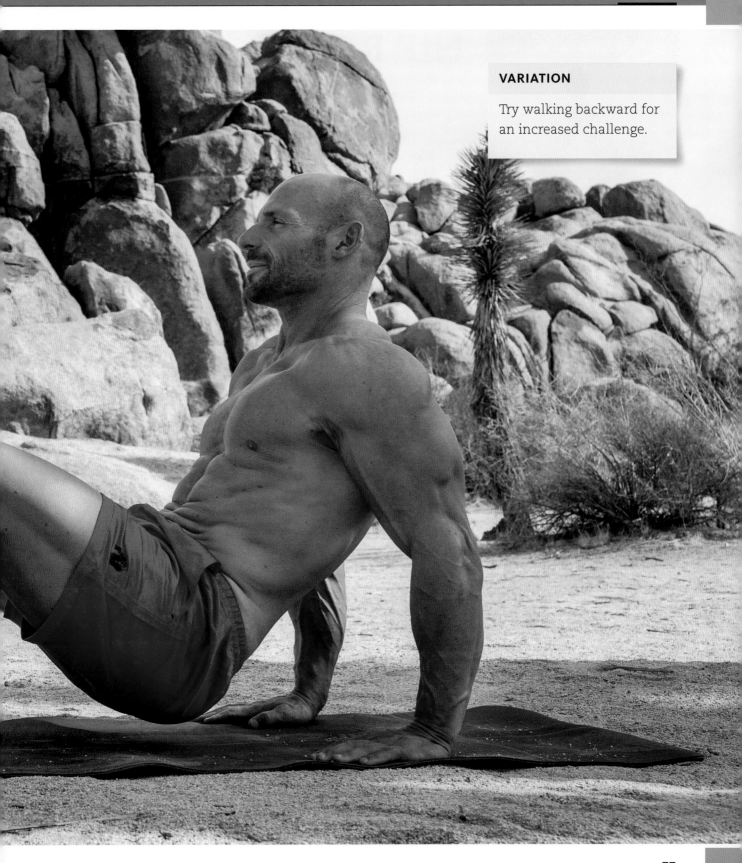

VARIATION

Try walking backward for an increased challenge.

PRIMARY MUSCLE ACTION

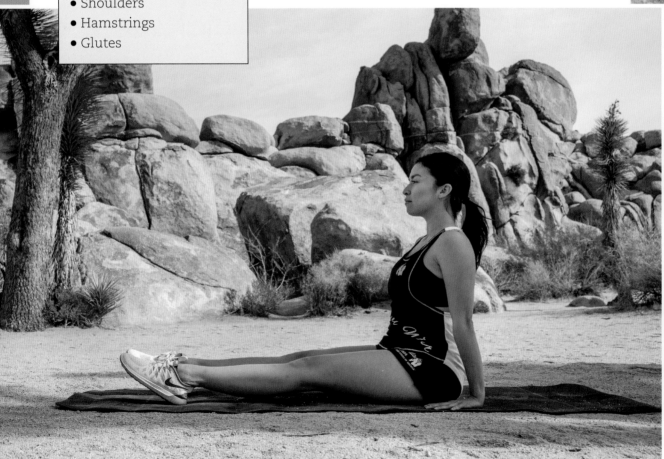

- Triceps
- Shoulders
- Hamstrings
- Glutes

HIP RAISER

PROGRESSION

1 Sit upright with your legs straight in front of you and your arms at your sides, palms down.

2 Push through your heels and palms while raising your pelvis upward until your legs are bent to a 90-degree angle and your body is largely a straight line.

3 Allow your head to float backward as you squeeze your glutes, then lower, and complete 15–20 repetitions.

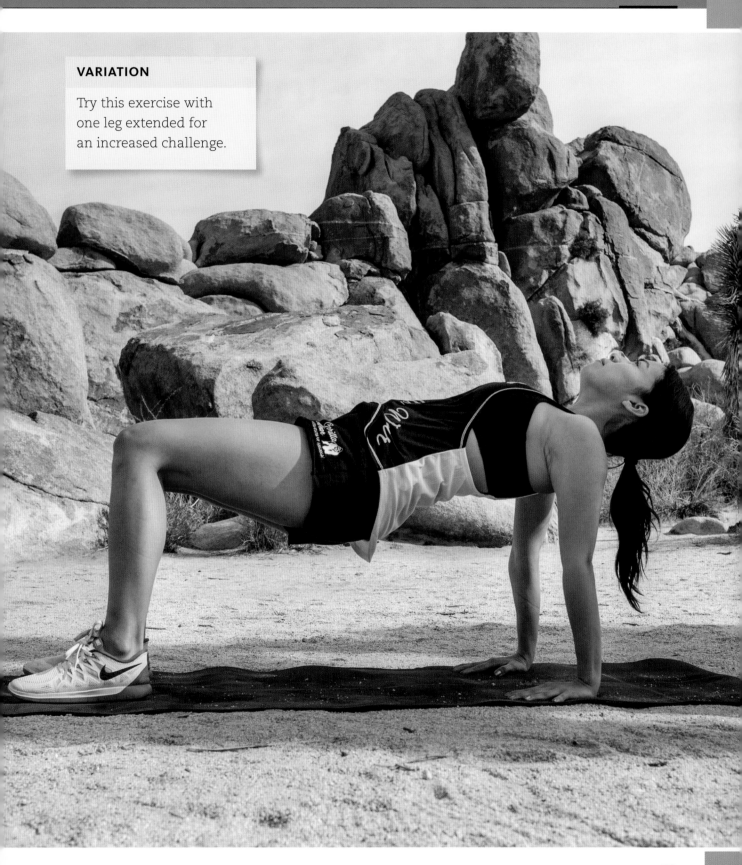

VARIATION

Try this exercise with one leg extended for an increased challenge.

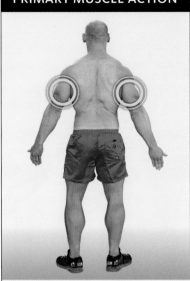

PRIMARY MUSCLE ACTION

- Triceps
- Core

SURFACE TRICEPS EXTENSION

PROGRESSION

1 Grasp a stable surface with your arms extended and your body in a straight line while on your toes.

2 Bend your arms at the elbows until your head is next to your hands, then push yourself back up to the starting position until your arms are locked.

3 Keep your elbows in and your core tight throughout the exercise, as you complete 15–20 repetitions.

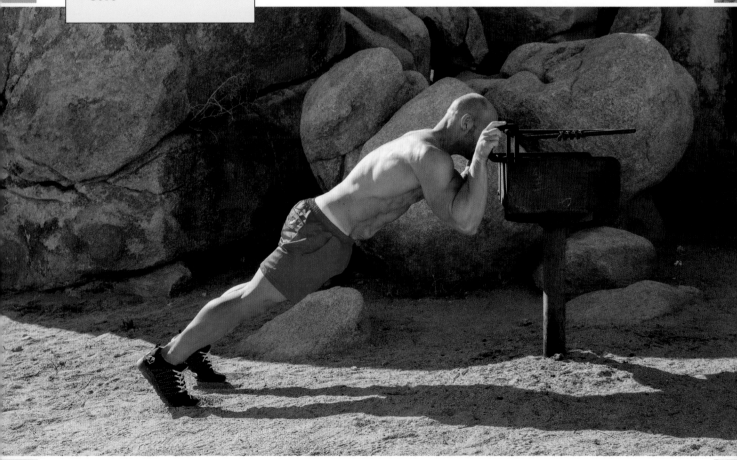

VARIATION

Try this exercise with one leg raised behind you for an increased challenge.

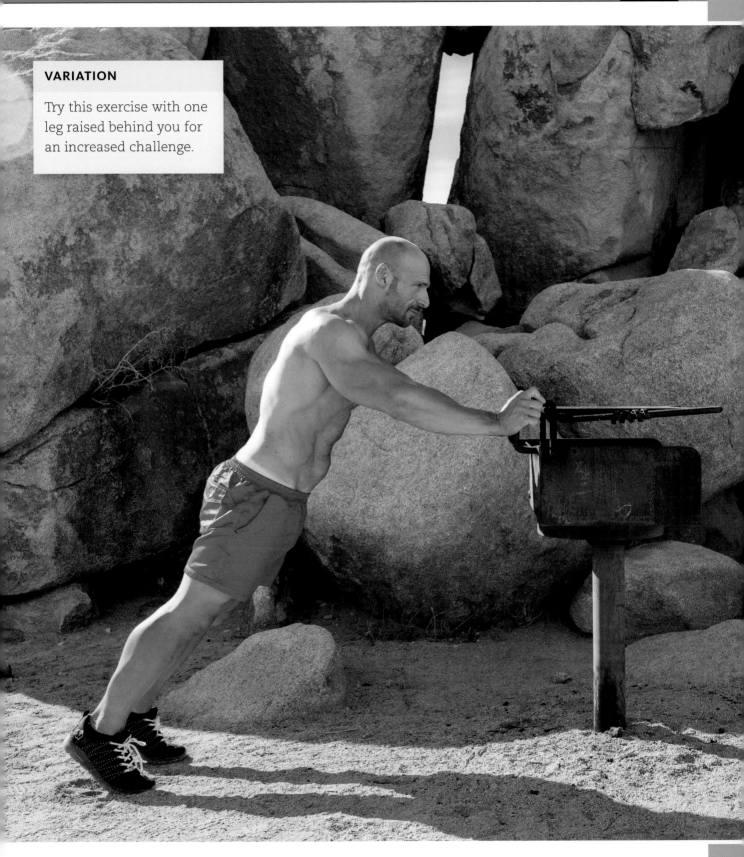

PRIMARY MUSCLE ACTION

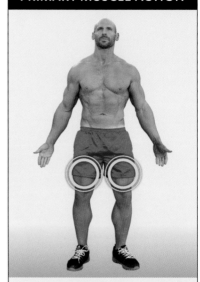

- Quadriceps
- Glutes
- Hamstrings

WALL SQUAT

PROGRESSION

1 Stand against a stable surface with your upper back touching it and your legs placed ahead in front so you are leaning back at an angle.

2 Cross your arms and bend at the knees until your thighs are parallel to the ground.

3 Push through your heels as you stand, and complete 15–20 repetitions.

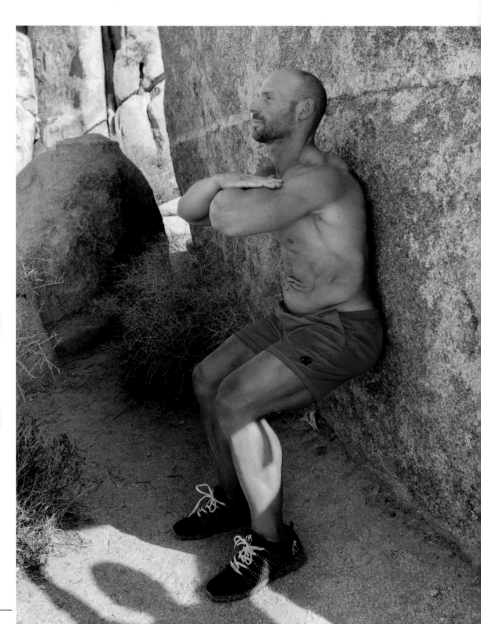

VARIATION

Try this exercise with one leg extended for an increased challenge.

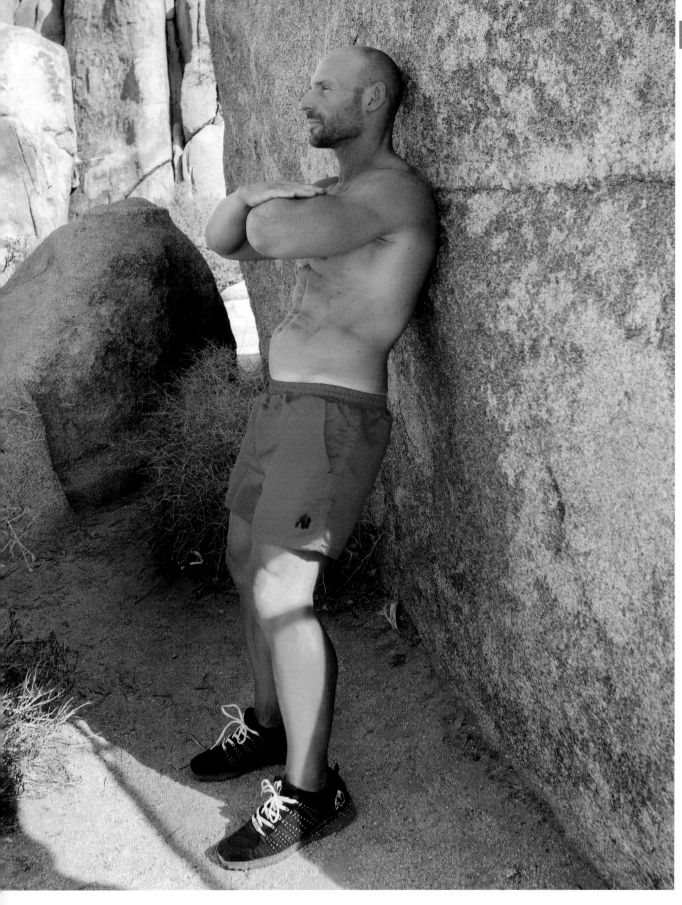

SHRIMP SQUAT

PROGRESSION

PRIMARY MUSCLE ACTION

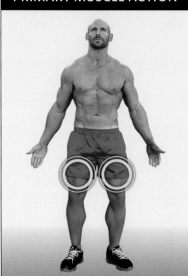

- Quadriceps
- Hamstrings
- Glutes
- Tibia

1 In a standing position, bend one leg back and hold your toes with one hand while outstretching your opposite arm in front for support.

2 Bend the standing leg slightly, then squat down until your thigh is nearly parallel to the ground.

3 Push through the heel as you return to the starting position.

4 Complete 10–12 repetitions, then switch legs.

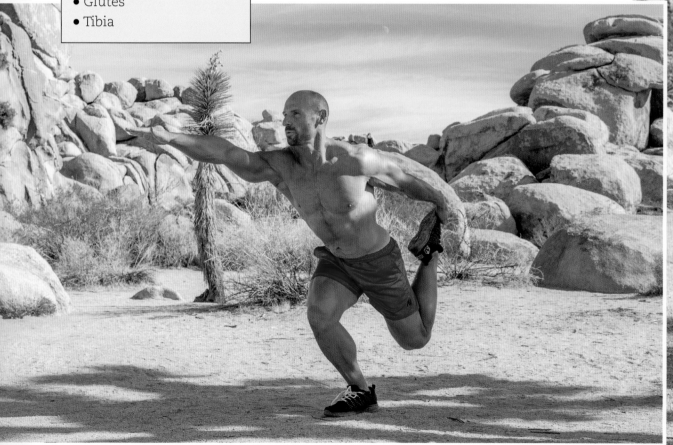

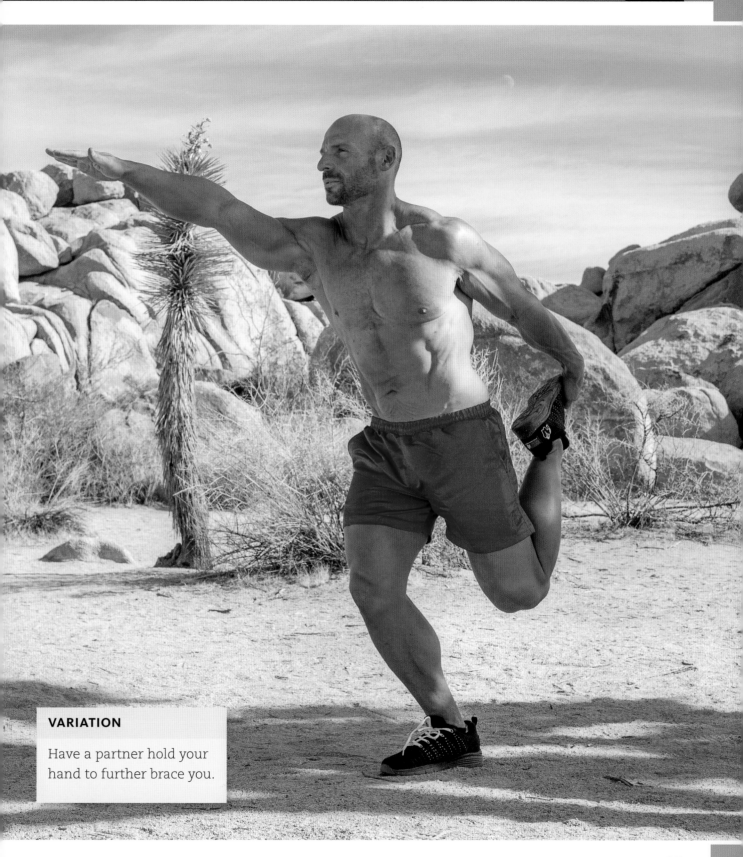

VARIATION

Have a partner hold your hand to further brace you.

PRIMARY MUSCLE ACTION

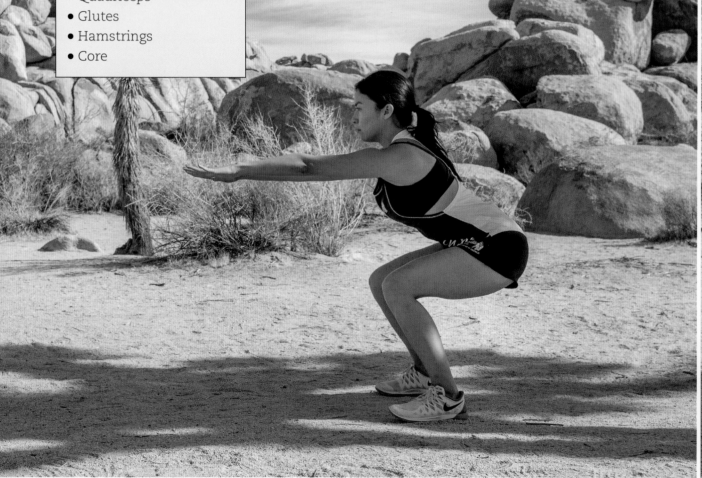

- Quadriceps
- Glutes
- Hamstrings
- Core

SQUAT

PROGRESSION

1 Stand with your feet shoulder-width apart and your arms bent in front of you.

2 Bend at the knees, sticking your rear out as you descend, until your thighs are parallel to the ground. At the same time, extend your arms in front of you.

3 Return to the starting position while pushing through your heels and drawing your arms back in, and complete 15–20 repetitions.

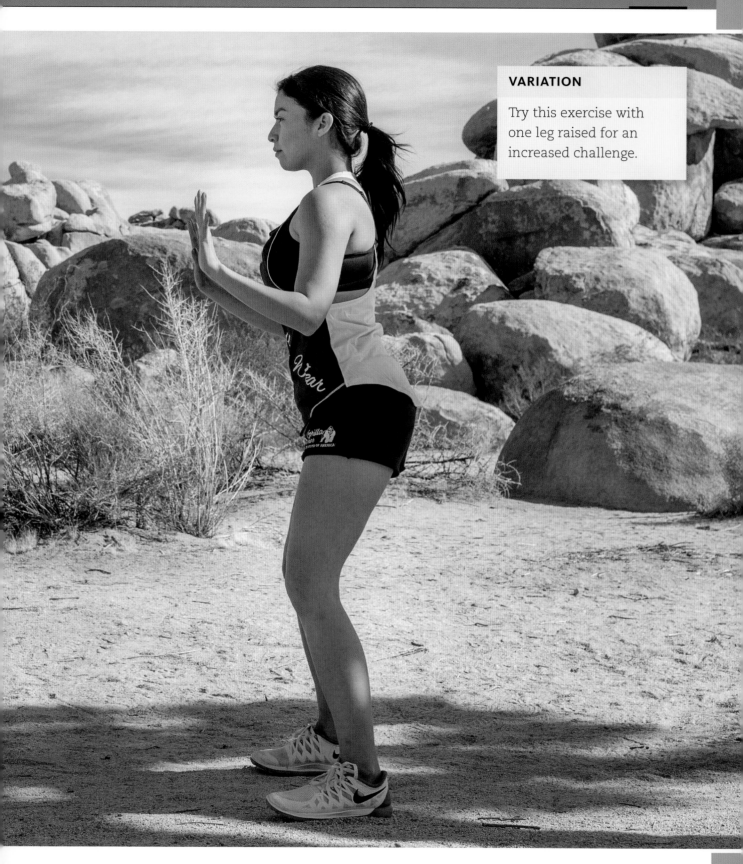

VARIATION

Try this exercise with one leg raised for an increased challenge.

PRIMARY MUSCLE ACTION

SINGLE-LEG BRIDGE

PROGRESSION

1 Lie back with both legs bent and your arms at your sides.

2 Push through one heel as you simultaneously raise your pelvis off the floor and extend the other leg straight up.

3 Squeeze your glutes, lower, and complete 15–20 repetitions, then switch to the other leg.

- Glutes
- Hamstrings
- Quadriceps
- Core

VARIATION

Make this exercise easier by bending the rising extended leg.

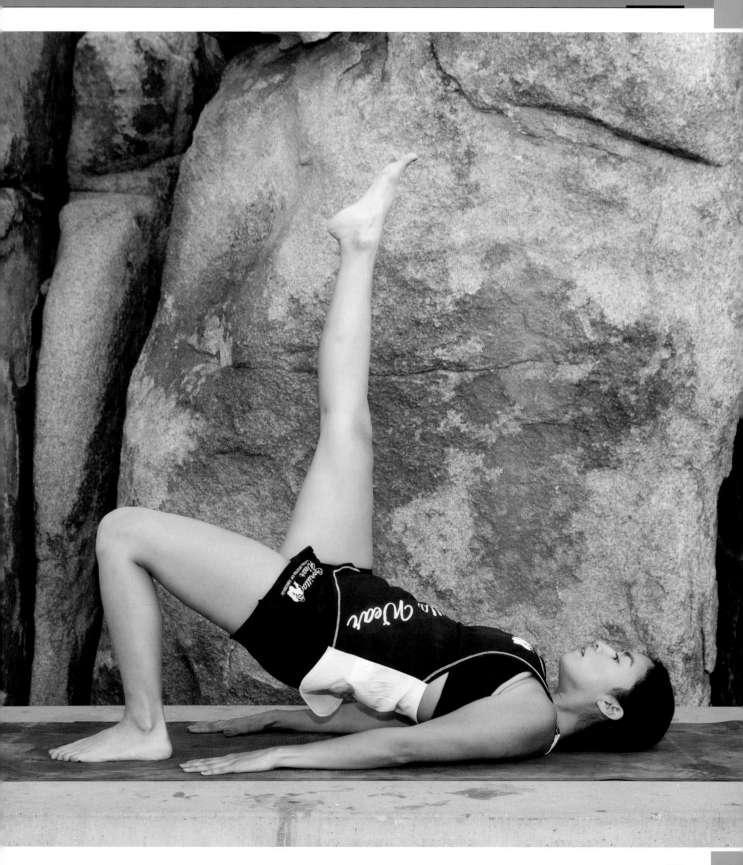

PRIMARY MUSCLE ACTION

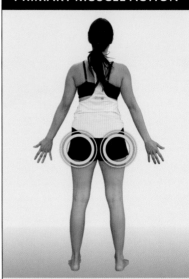

- Glutes
- Hamstrings
- Quadriceps

BUTT KICKS

PROGRESSION

1 In a standing position, begin jogging in place while bringing your heels behind you to tap your glutes.

2 Continue for 50 repetitions per leg.

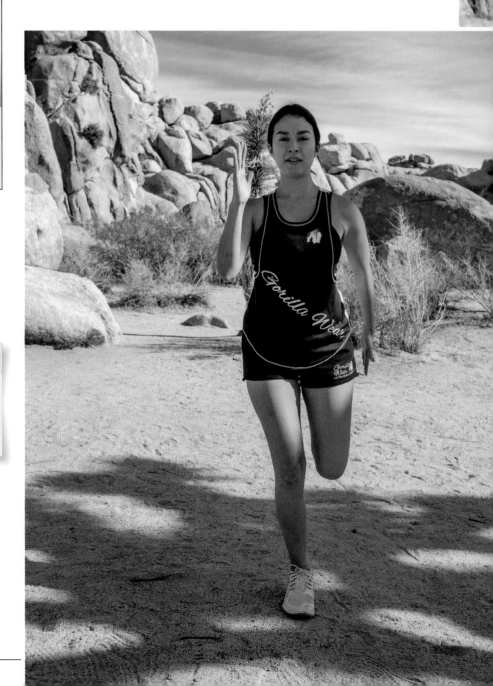

VARIATION

Try this exercise while jogging forward for an increased challenge.

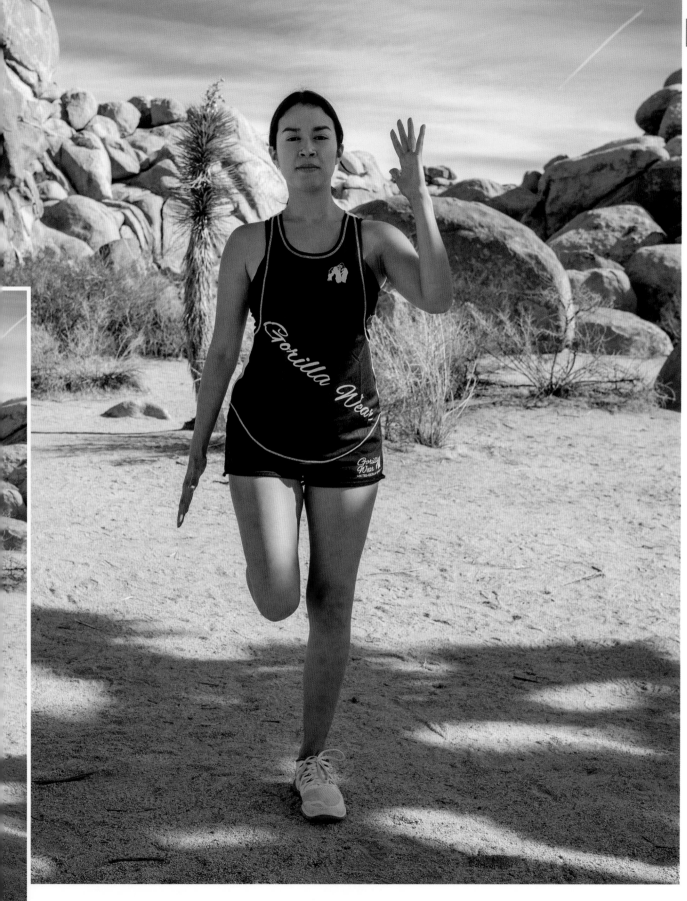

PRIMARY MUSCLE ACTION

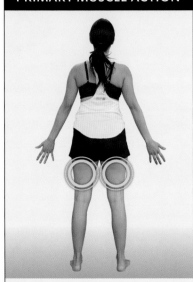

- Hamstrings
- Core

T-STAND

PROGRESSION

1 Stand with your arms at your sides and your feet close together.

2 Lean forward slowly, allowing your arms to dangle as you raise one leg straight behind you, keeping your head raised.

3 Return to the starting position in a fluid, controlled manner.

4 Complete 15–20 repetitions, then switch legs.

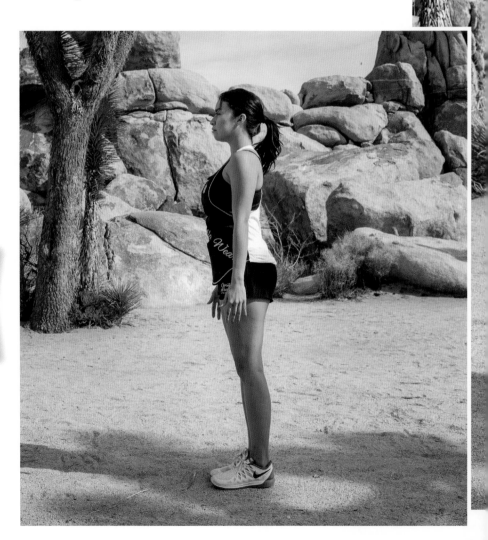

VARIATION

Make this exercise easier by supporting yourself against a sturdy object.

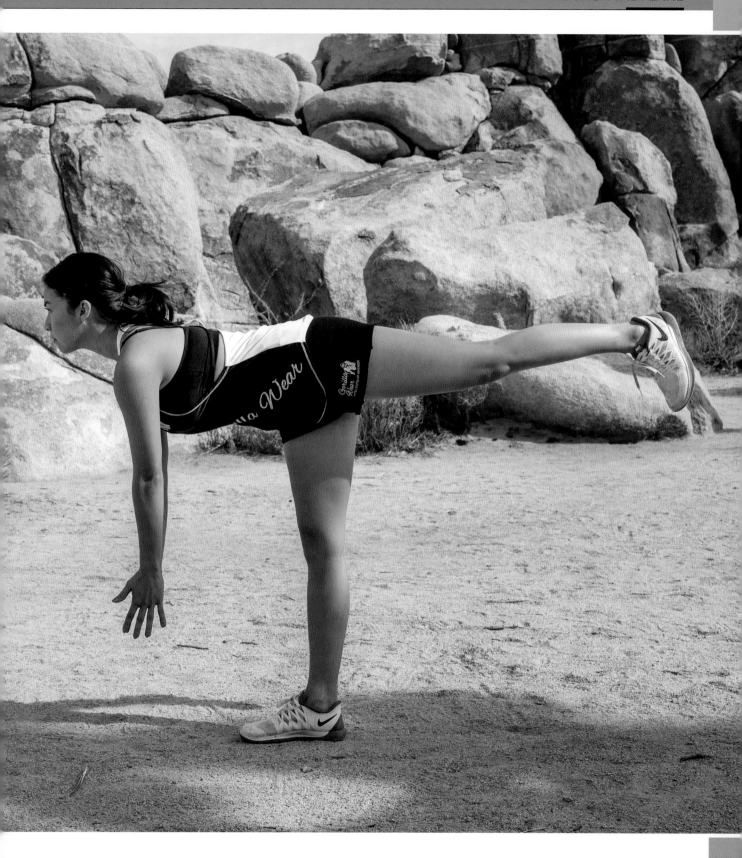

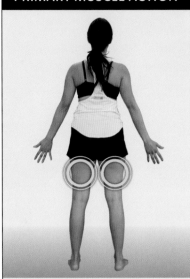

PRIMARY MUSCLE ACTION

- Hamstrings
- Chest
- Deltoids

HAM SANDWICH

PROGRESSION

1 Place a mat on the ground and kneel on it while maintaining a straight back.

2 Have a partner hold your ankles to keep you in place.

3 Fall forward in a controlled fashion using your hamstrings like brakes, with your hands up to support you as your chest nears the ground.

4 Explode back upward again using your hamstrings, and complete 12–15 repetitions.

VARIATION

Try this exercise with one hand up for an increased challenge.

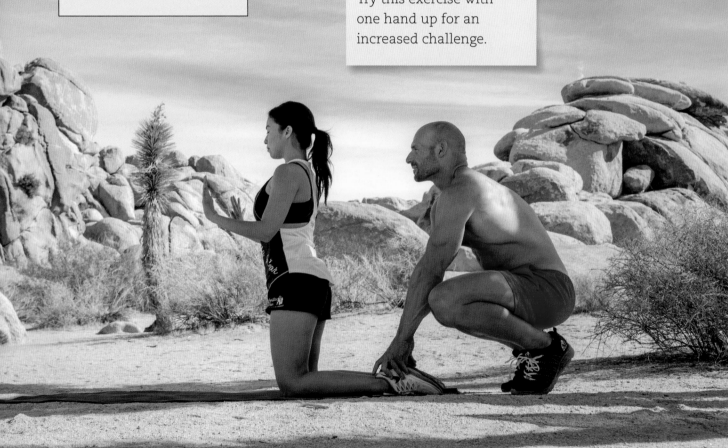

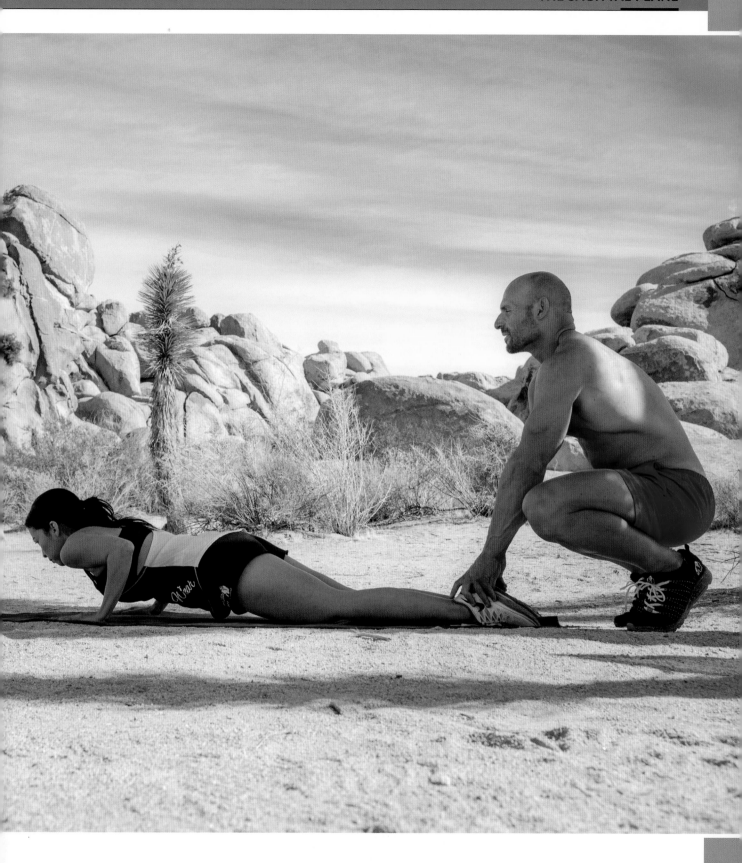

PRIMARY MUSCLE ACTION

- Calves

STANDING CALF RAISE

PROGRESSION

1 Stand facing a sturdy vertical surface, and lean into it using your hands for support.

2 Rise up on your toes, flexing your calf muscles at the top.

3 Lower, and complete 15–20 repetitions.

VARIATION

Try this exercise while standing on one leg for an increased challenge.

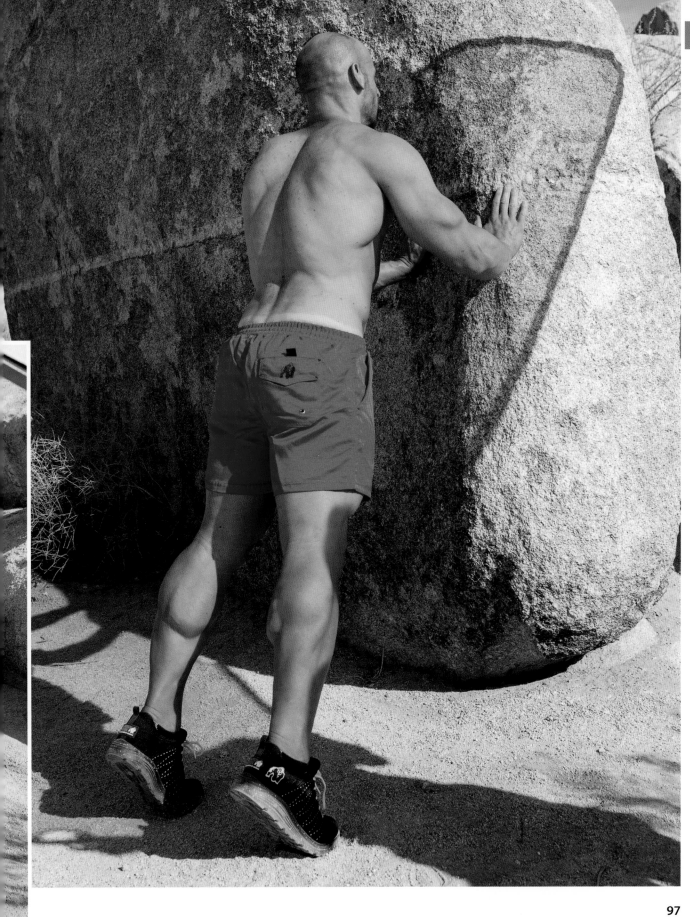

PRIMARY MUSCLE ACTION

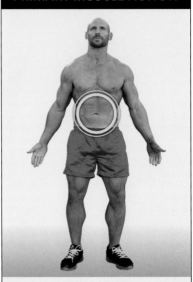

- Abdominals
- Spinal Erectors

DOUBLE LEG LIFT

PROGRESSION

1 Lie on your back with your hands tucked slightly under your glutes and your legs extended.

2 Raise your legs, keeping them slightly bent to alleviate lower-back stress.

3 Lower to just short of the ground, and complete 20 repetitions.

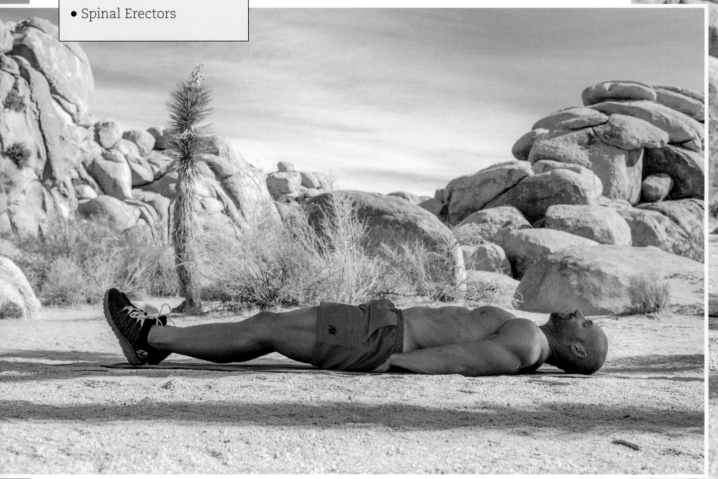

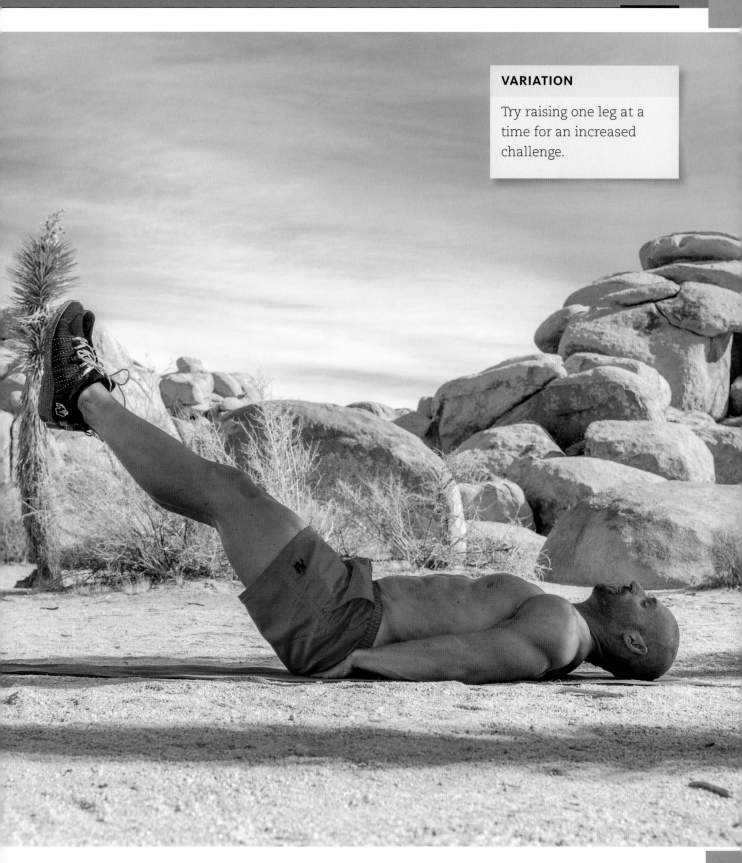

VARIATION

Try raising one leg at a time for an increased challenge.

PRIMARY MUSCLE ACTION

• Abdominals

MEDICINE-BALL SIT-UP

PROGRESSION

1 Lie on your back with your legs bent while holding a medicine ball near your chest.

2 Rise upward through your torso toward your legs while holding the medicine ball in place.

3 Lower, and complete 20 repetitions.

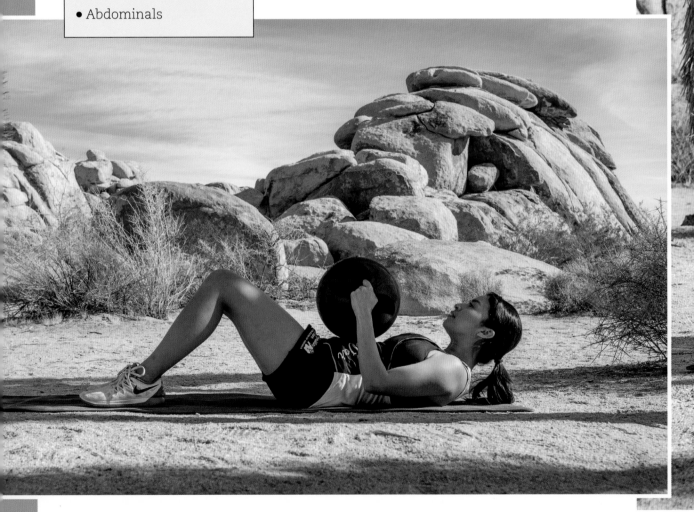

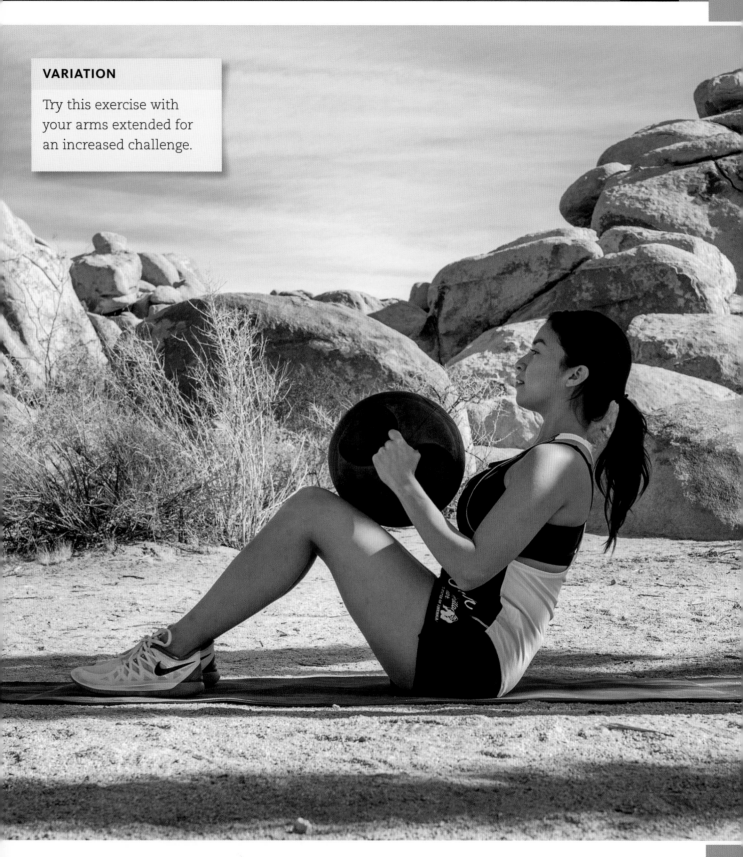

VARIATION

Try this exercise with your arms extended for an increased challenge.

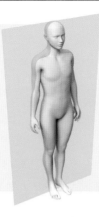

THE FRONTAL PLANE divides the body into front and back halves. Lateral side movements along this plane are considered frontal.

PRIMARY MUSCLE ACTION

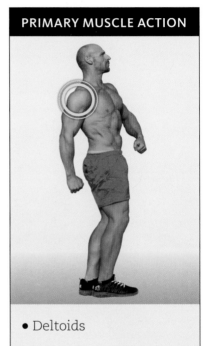

• Deltoids

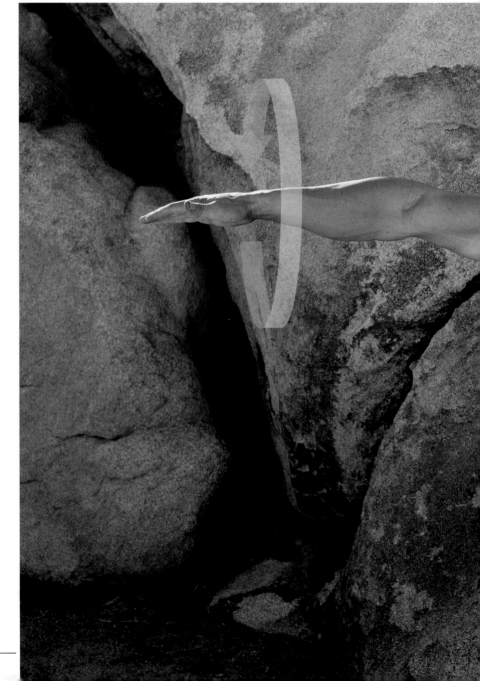

ARM ROTATION

PROGRESSION

1 Stand with your arms outstretched and make large or small rotations, completing 50 repetitions.

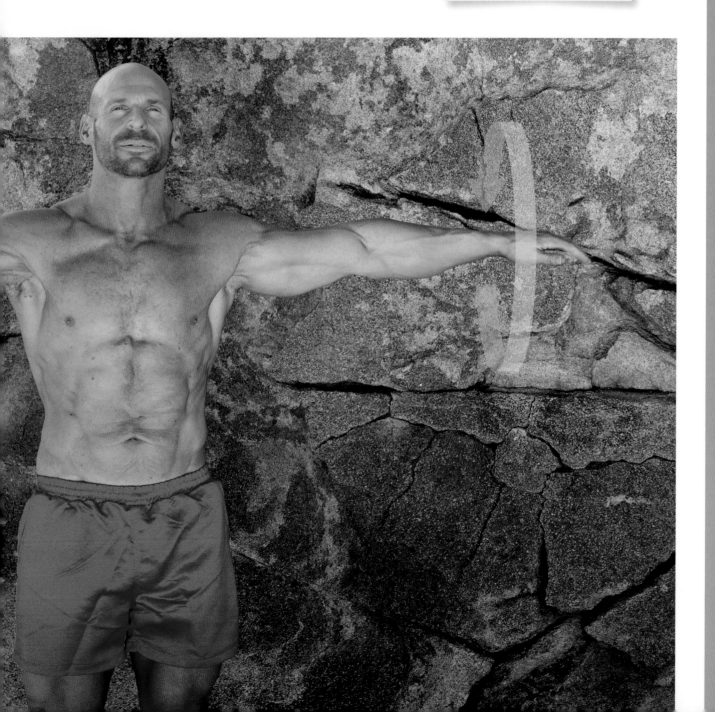

PRIMARY MUSCLE ACTION

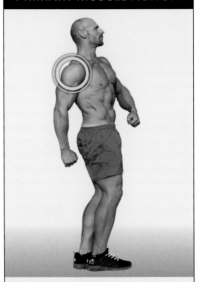

- Deltoids
- Hip Flexors
- Obliques
- Intercostals

HIP-UP

PROGRESSION

1 Lie on one side, propped up on your forearm, with your other hand on your hip, your head up, and one extended leg on top of the other.

2 Raise your pelvis so your body becomes a straight line, hold for a few seconds, lower, and complete 12–15 repetitions.

3 Switch to the other side.

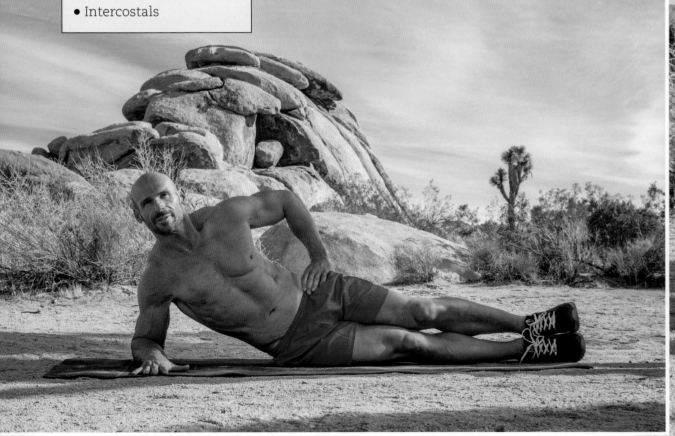

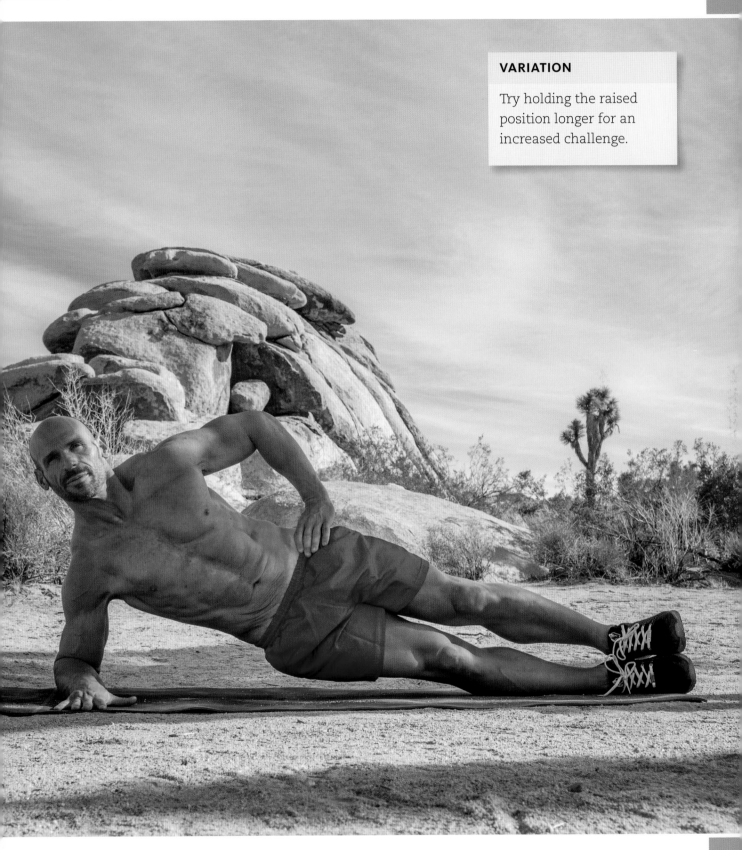

VARIATION

Try holding the raised position longer for an increased challenge.

PRIMARY MUSCLE ACTION

THUMBS-UP

PROGRESSION

1 Lie face down with both arms outstretched and your thumbs pointed upward.

2 Raise your head and shoulders off the ground while lifting your arms as high as you can.

3 Hold for a few seconds, and complete 12–15 repetitions.

- Rear Deltoids
- Spinal Erectors

VARIATION

While in the upward contracted position, try rotating your thumbs forward for an increased challenge.

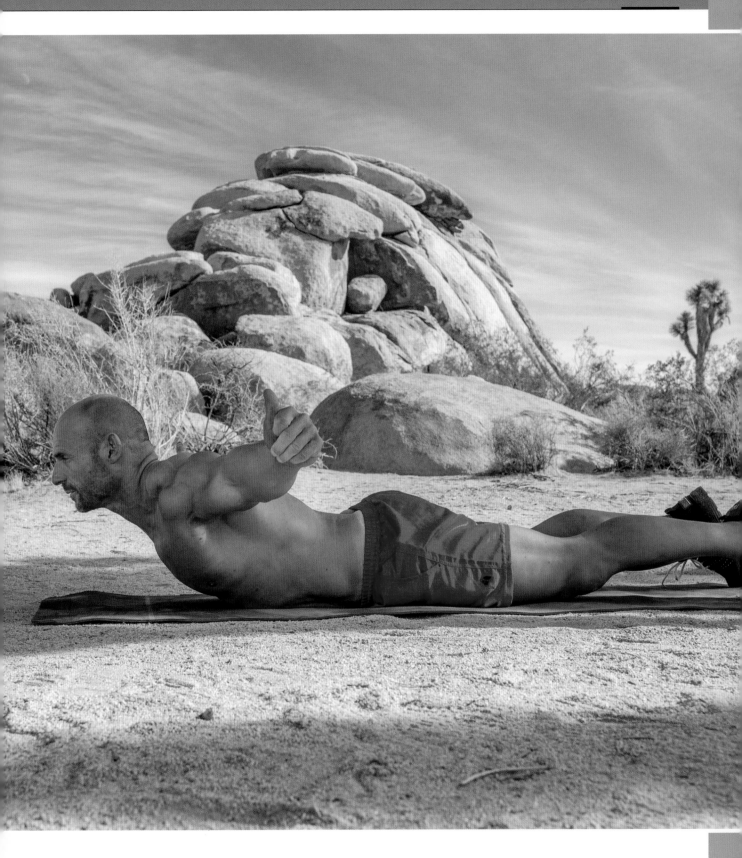

PRIMARY MUSCLE ACTION

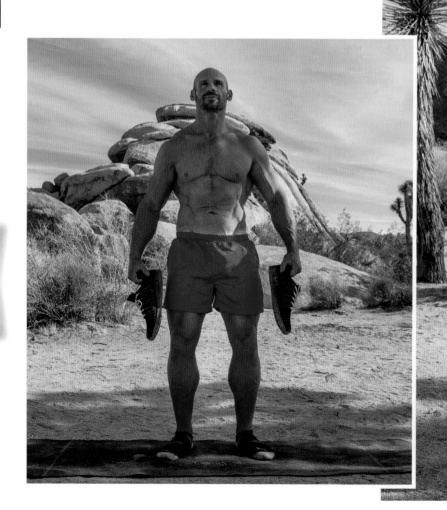

• Medial Deltoids

LATERAL SHOULDER RAISE

PROGRESSION

1 Start from a standing position, with your arms down at your sides, holding a pair of sneakers.

2 Raise your arms outward until they are parallel to the ground.

3 Lower, and complete 15–20 repetitions.

VARIATION

Try this exercise while standing on one leg for an increased challenge.

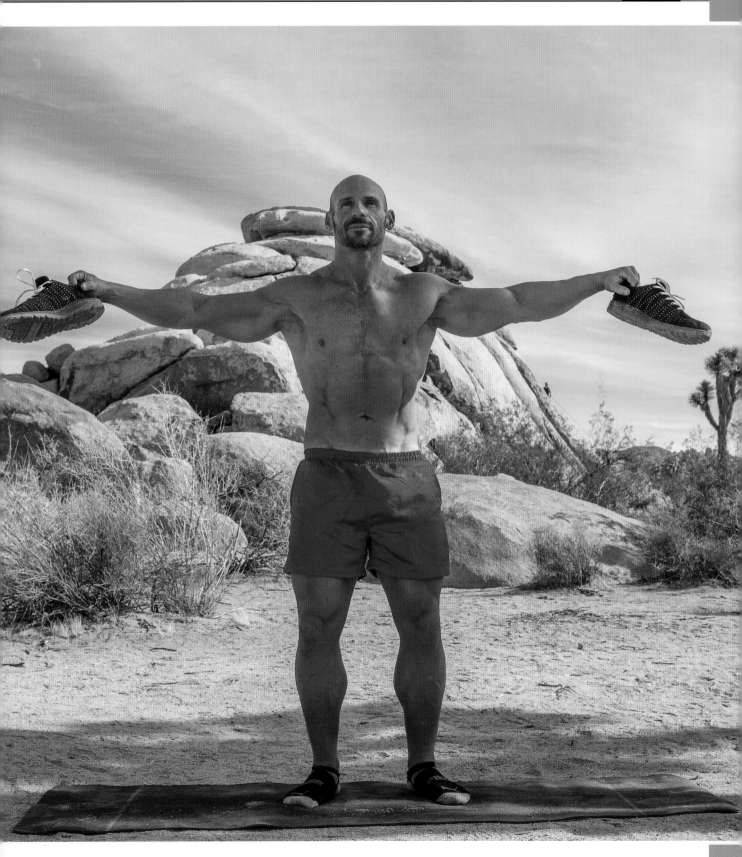

PRIMARY MUSCLE ACTION

• Posterior Deltoids

BENT-OVER LATERAL RAISE

PROGRESSION

1 Start in a bent-forward position, while maintaining a flat back and holding a pair of sneakers down in front of you with slightly bent arms.

2 Raise your arms directly to your sides in a reverse hugging motion, until you can squeeze your shoulder blades together.

3 Lower, and complete 15–20 repetitions.

VARIATION

Try this exercise while standing on one leg for an increased challenge.

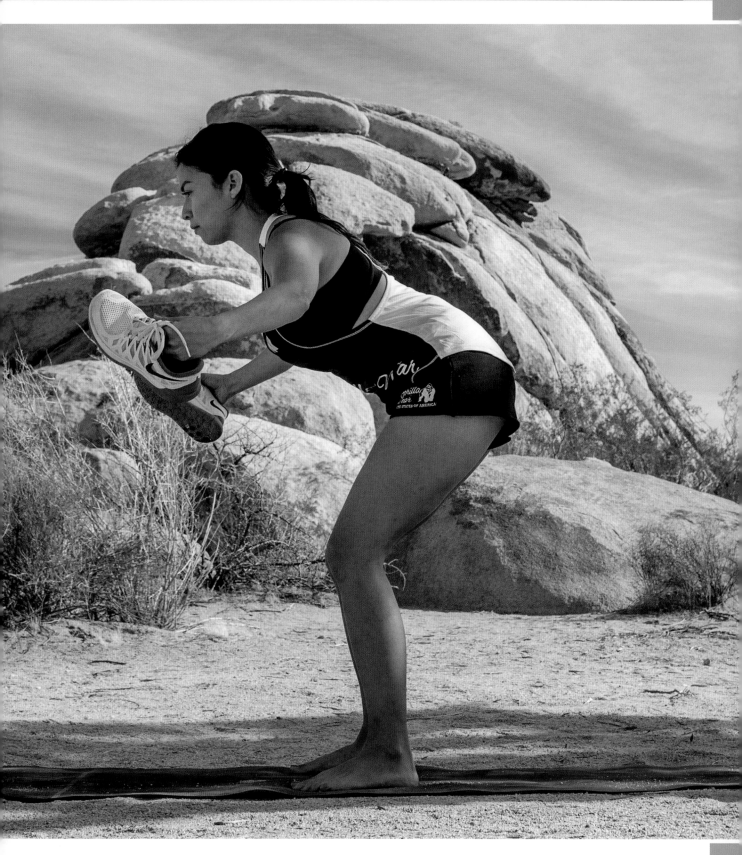

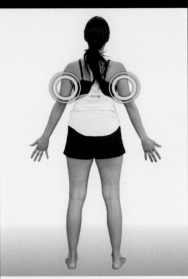

PRIMARY MUSCLE ACTION

- Triceps
- Obliques

SIDE TRICEPS EXTENSION

PROGRESSION

1 While lying on your right side in a straight line, cross your right arm over your chest, placing your right hand on your left shoulder. Plant your left hand on the ground, with fingers pointing toward your chest.

2 While keeping your body a straight line, push your upper body off the ground until your planted arm is extended.

3 Complete 12–15 repetitions, then switch to the other side.

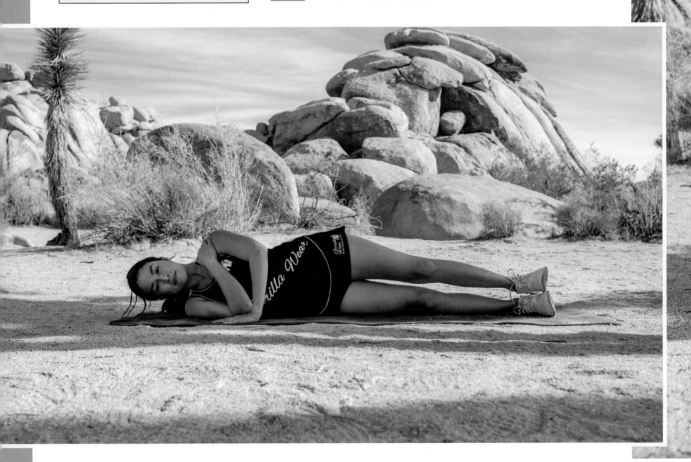

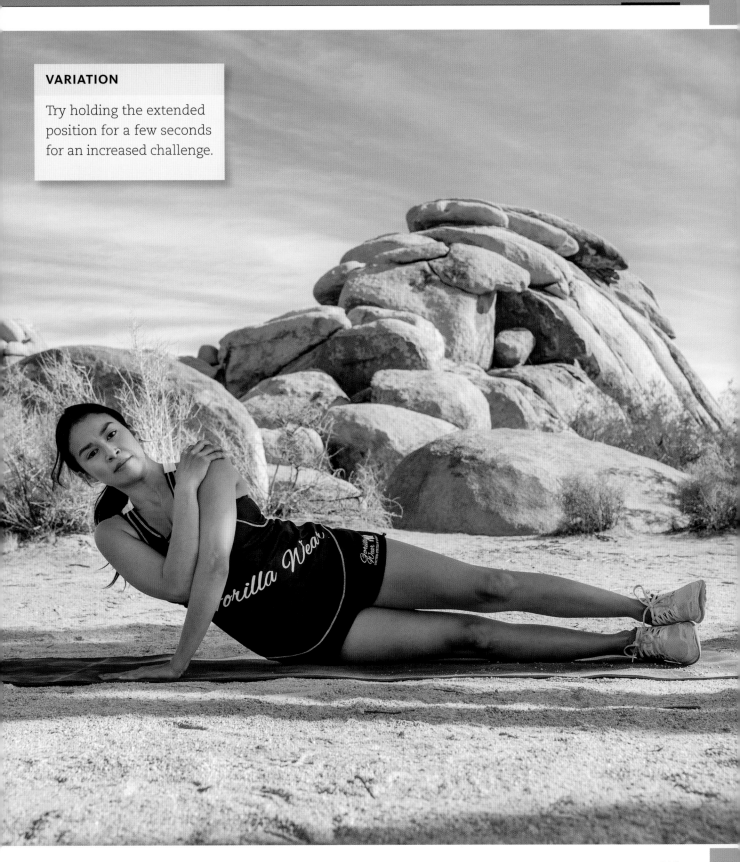

VARIATION

Try holding the extended position for a few seconds for an increased challenge.

PRIMARY MUSCLE ACTION

- Quadriceps
- Hamstrings
- Glutes

SIDE LUNGE

PROGRESSION

1 Begin in a standing position, with your legs apart and your arms extended downward.

2 Keeping your torso facing forward throughout, lunge to the right by bending the right leg while keeping the left leg straight.

3 Return to the starting position, complete 12–15 repetitions, then continue with the opposite leg.

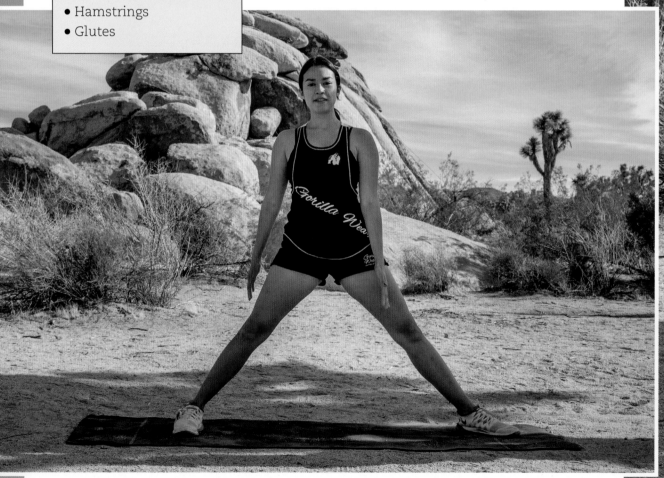

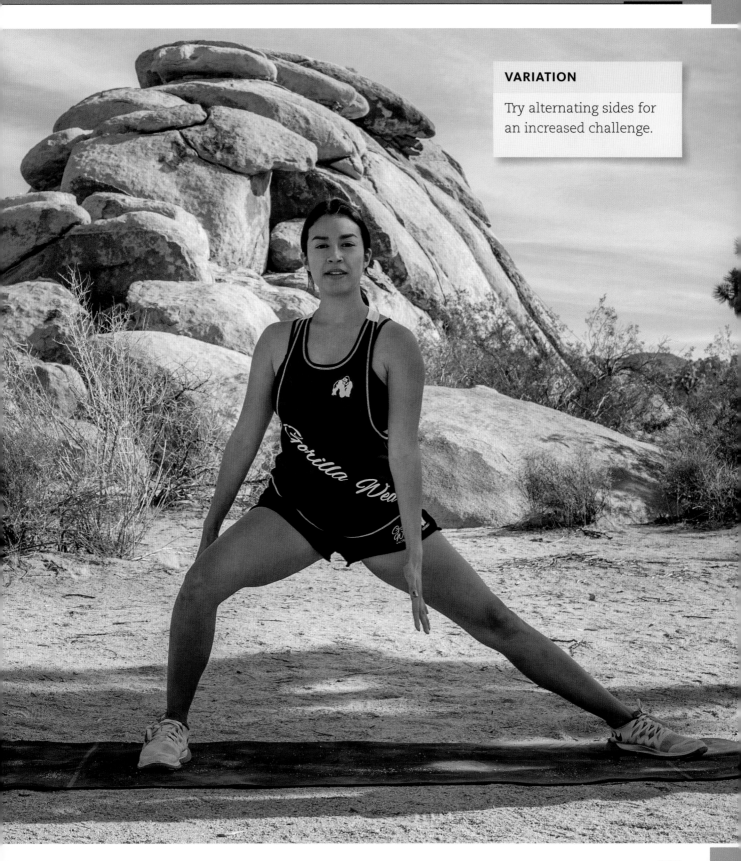

VARIATION

Try alternating sides for an increased challenge.

PRIMARY MUSCLE ACTION

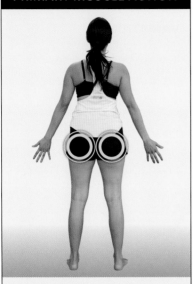

- Glutes
- Inner Thighs
- Hamstrings
- Core
- Calves

SQUAT AND SIDE KICK

PROGRESSION

1 In a standing position—with feet shoulder-width apart, knees bent, rear propped out, and fists up—squat downward while keeping your core tight.

2 As you return to the starting position, extend one leg out to the side until it's parallel to the ground.

3 Complete 12–15 repetitions, then continue with the other leg.

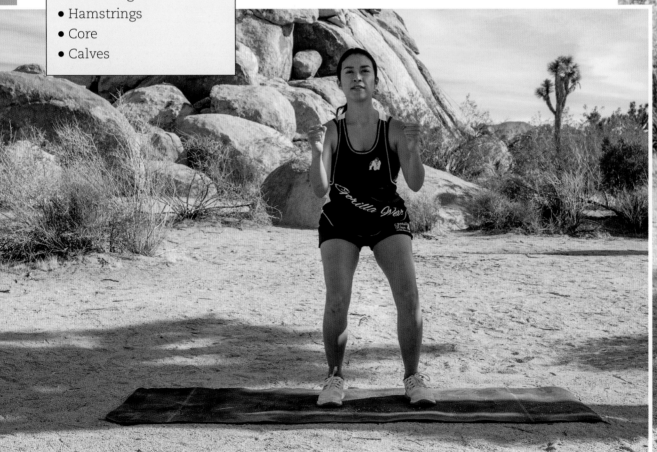

VARIATION

Try alternating sides for an increased challenge.

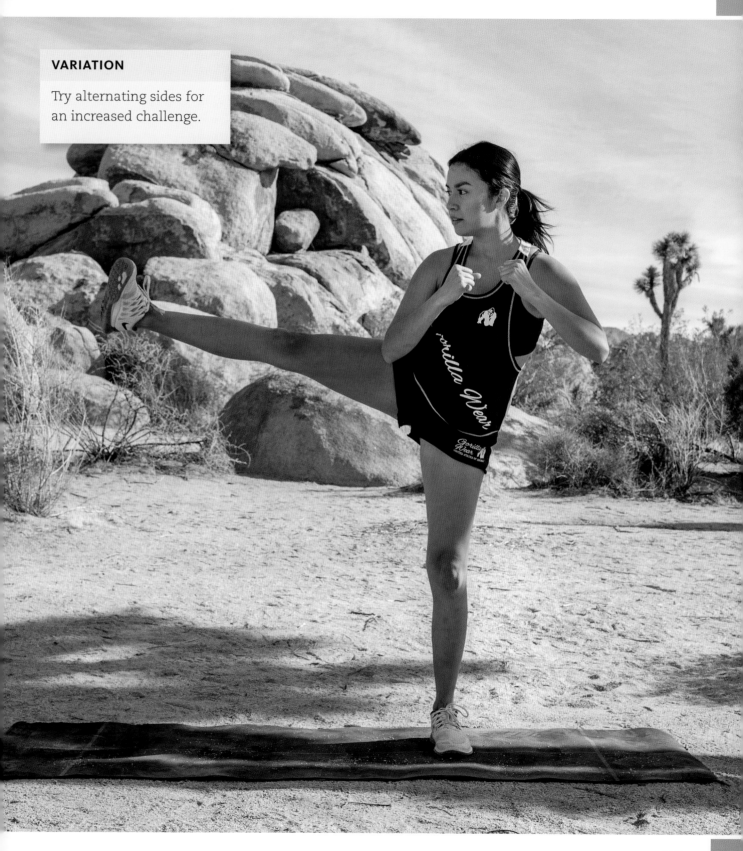

PRIMARY MUSCLE ACTION

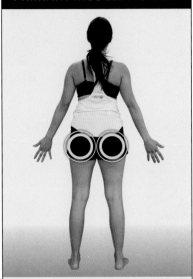

- Glutes
- Hip Flexors
- Spinal Erectors

STANDING SIDE LEG LIFT

PROGRESSION

1 Stand with your feet together, and place your left hand on a solid surface.

2 Raise your right leg out to the side, foot flexed, while maintaining a forward-facing posture.

3 Contract your glutes, complete 15–20 repetitions, and switch to the opposite leg.

VARIATION

Try this exercise without any support for an increased challenge.

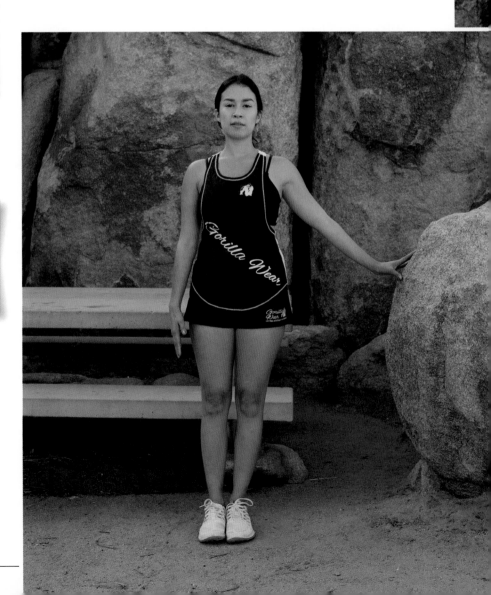

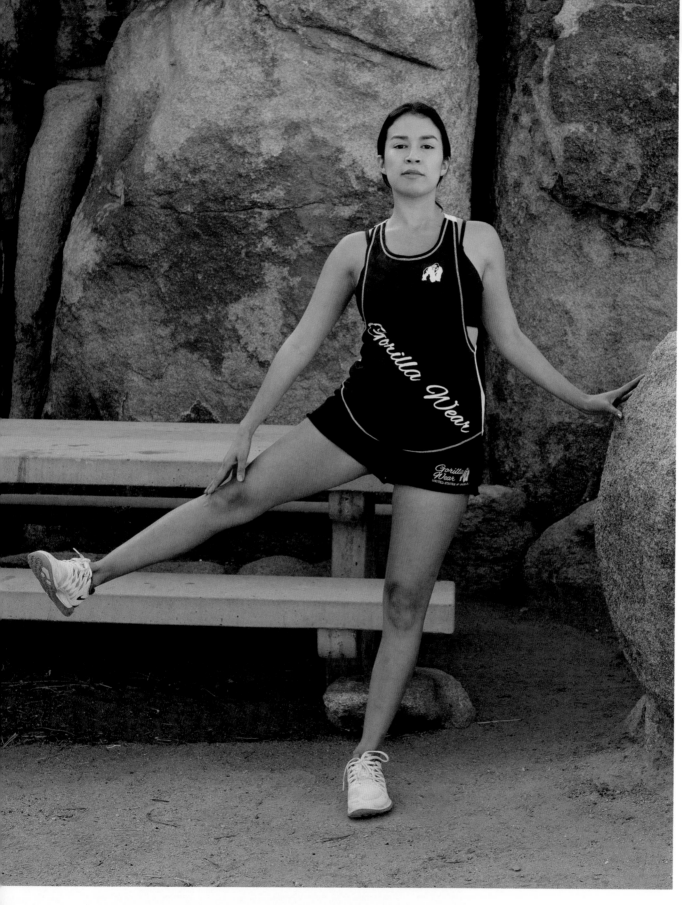

PRIMARY MUSCLE ACTION

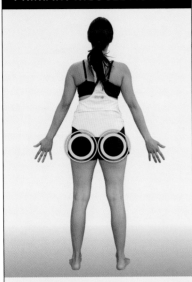

- Glutes
- Hamstrings
- Core
- Calves

KNEE TO SHOULDER
PROGRESSION

1 In a standing position, with your right arm raised overhead and your left hand on your hip, lift the right knee toward your shoulder while simultaneously lowering your raised arm until your elbow nearly touches the knee.

2 Lower, and complete 20–25 repetitions, then switch to the other side.

VARIATION

Try straightening the raised leg out to the side for an increased challenge.

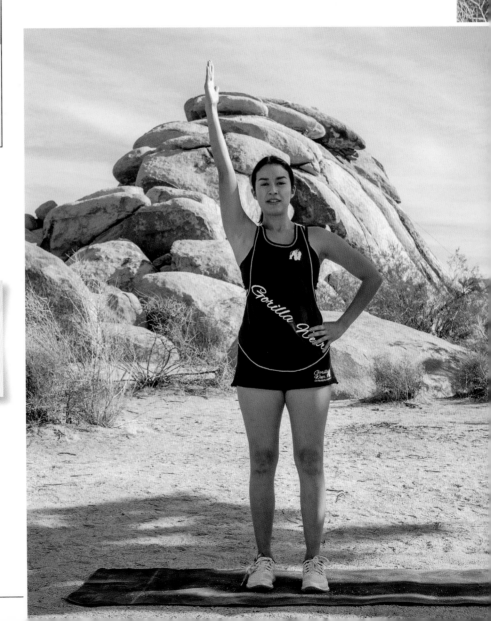

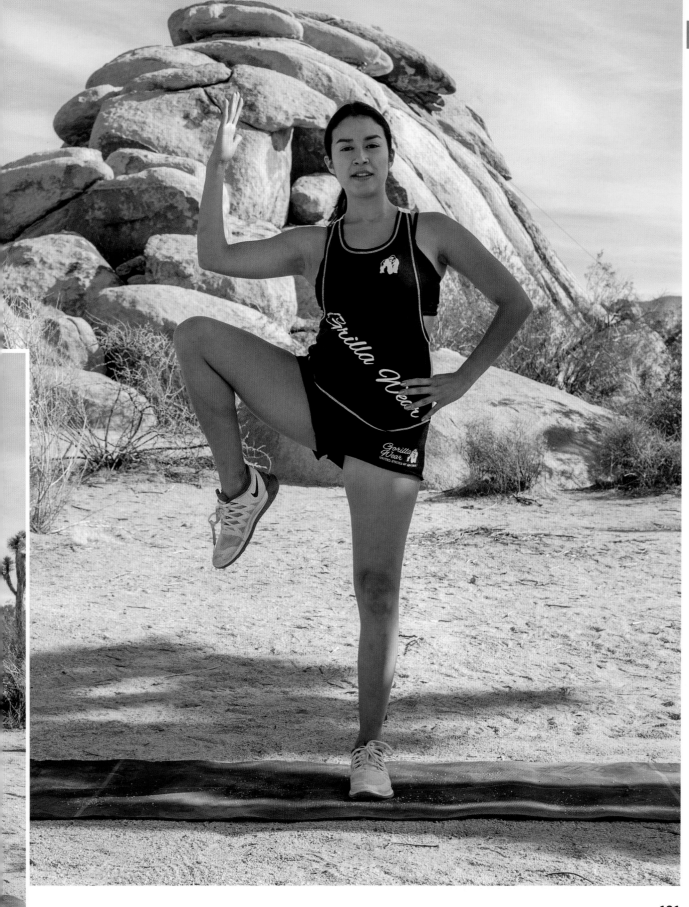

PRIMARY MUSCLE ACTION

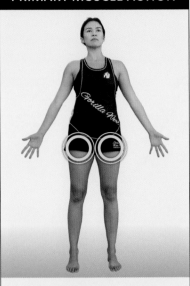

- Hip Flexors
- Obliques

BEACH SCISSORS

PROGRESSION

1 Lie on your side, propped up on your forearm, with your other hand on your hip, your head straight on, and one extended leg on top of the other.

2 Raise your free leg as high as you can, pause, lower, and complete 15–20 repetitions.

3 Switch to the other leg.

VARIATION

Try holding the extended position longer for an increased challenge.

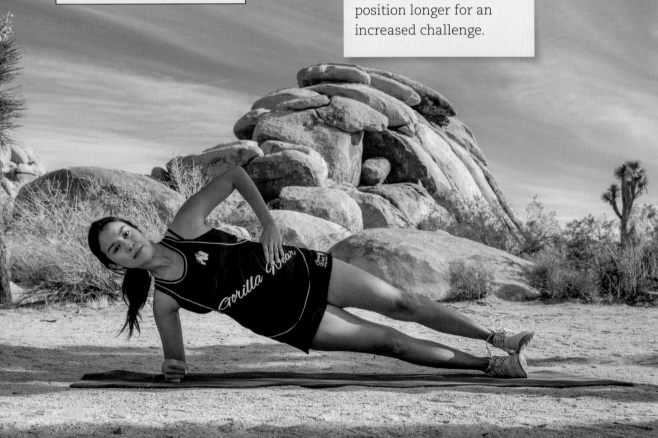

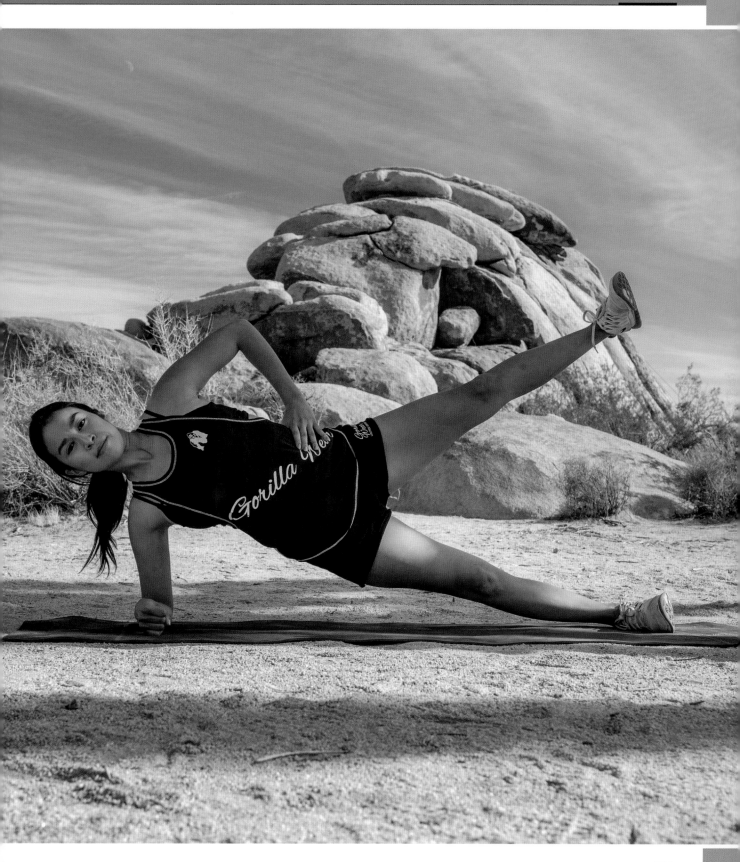

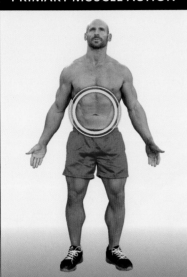

PRIMARY MUSCLE ACTION

- Core
- Triceps
- Deltoids

PLANK TAP

PROGRESSION

1 Begin in a push-up position.

2 Lift one hand while locked out in the top portion of the push-up, and touch your opposite shoulder.

3 Return to the starting position, and alternate sides for 15–20 repetitions.

VARIATION

Try holding the finished position for a few seconds for an increased challenge.

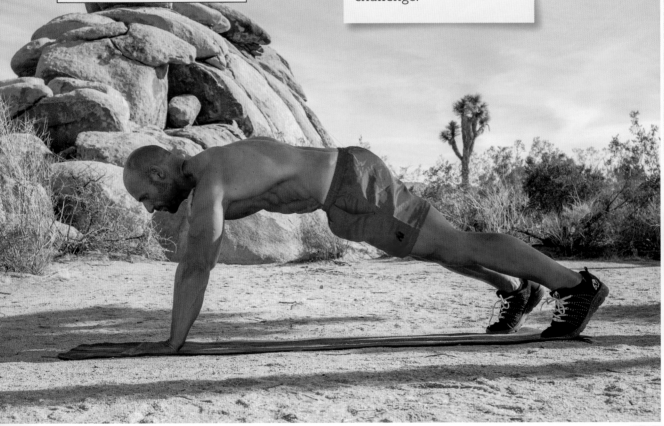

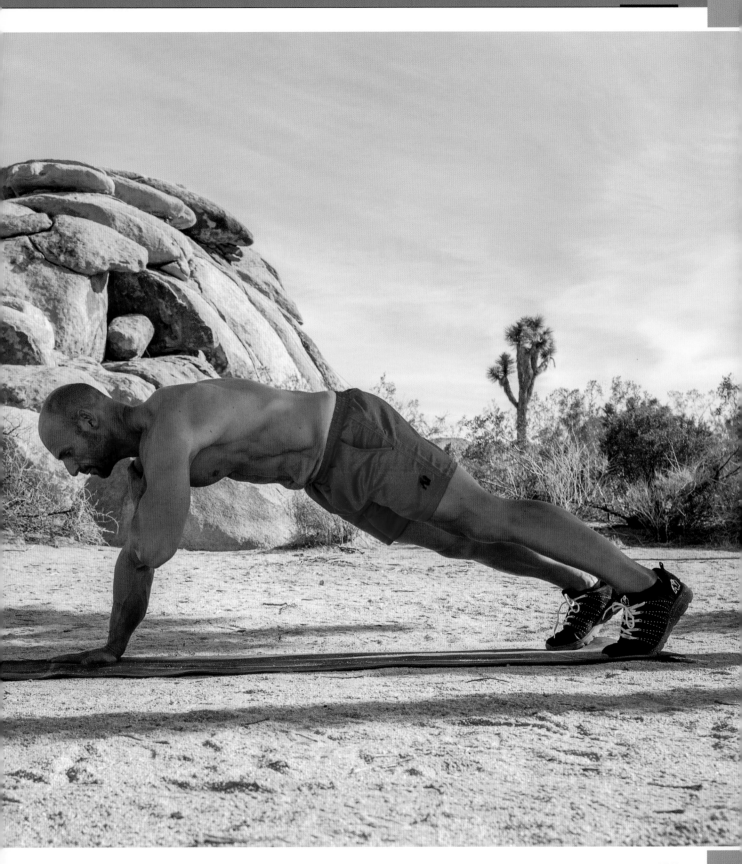

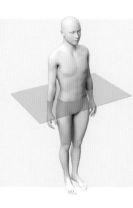

THE TRANSVERSE PLANE divides the body into upper and lower halves. Rotational movement along this plane is considered transverse.

PRIMARY MUSCLE ACTION

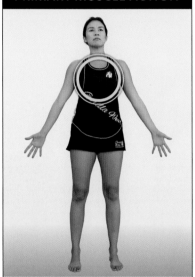

- Chest
- Deltoids
- Triceps
- Core
- Glutes

SPIDER-MAN PUSH-UP

PROGRESSION

1 Begin at the top of a standard push-up position.

2 As you start to lower, lift one foot off the ground and rotate that knee toward your shoulder.

3 Return to the starting position, and alternate for 15–20 repetitions per side.

VARIATION

Try bringing the opposite knee toward your shoulder for an increased challenge.

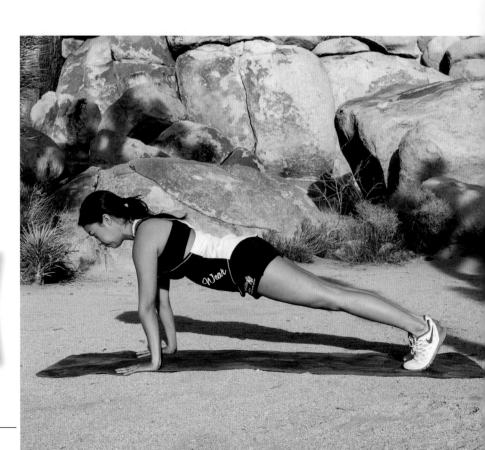

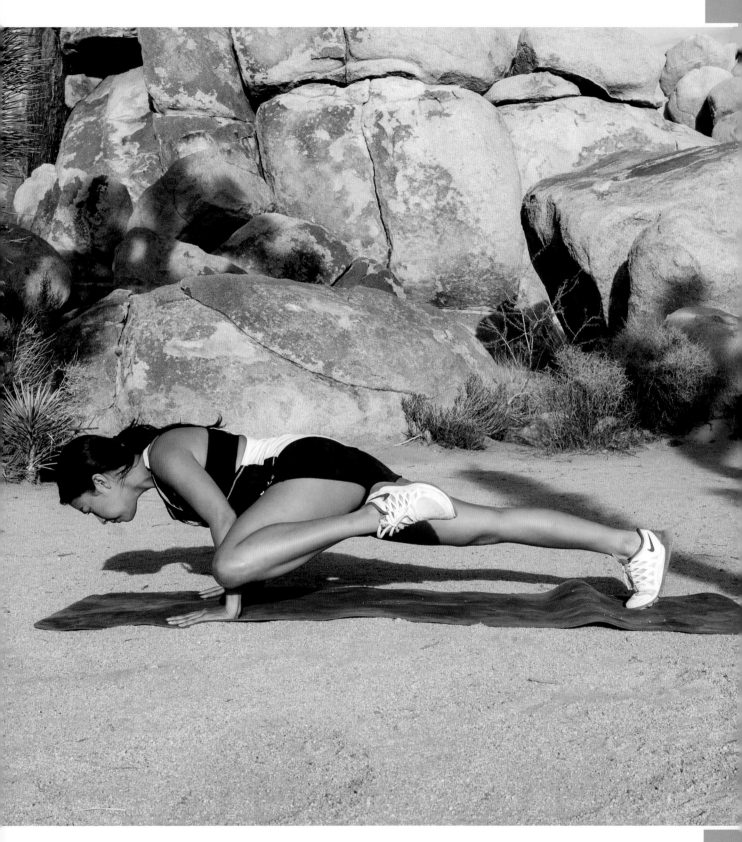

PRIMARY MUSCLE ACTION

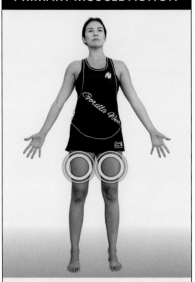

- Quadriceps
- Glutes
- Hamstrings
- Core

DIAGONAL MOUNTAIN CLIMBER

PROGRESSION

1 Begin at the top of a standard push-up position.

2 In rapid succession, bring one knee toward the opposite elbow and return to the starting point, then switch knees while keeping your hips down.

3 Alternate for 50 repetitions.

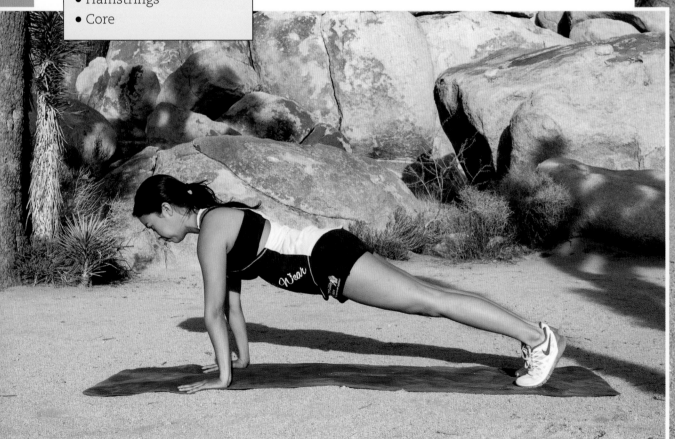

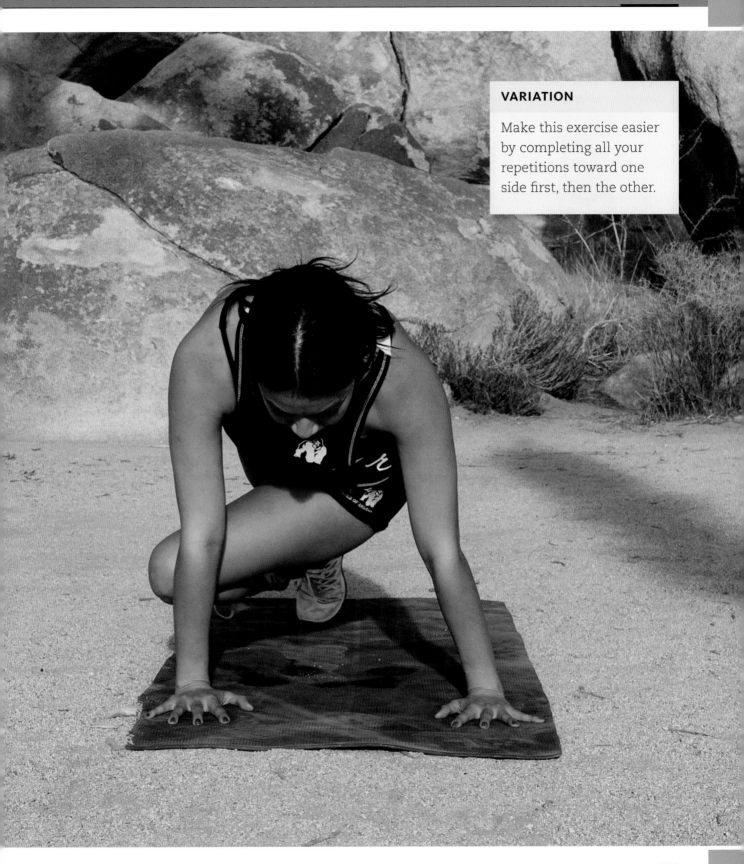

VARIATION

Make this exercise easier by completing all your repetitions toward one side first, then the other.

PRIMARY MUSCLE ACTION

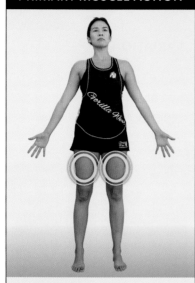

- Quadriceps
- Glutes
- Hamstrings
- Core

HINGING LUNGE

PROGRESSION

1 Begin in a leaning-forward position, with your right leg bent at 90 degrees in front of you and your left leg outstretched behind you.

2 Plant your left hand in front, and raise your right hand behind you.

3 Stand to lengthen your right leg as much as possible while you simultaneously turn your head to the same side.

4 Complete 12–15 repetitions, then switch sides.

VARIATION

Try this exercise without the stabilizing hand in front for an increased challenge.

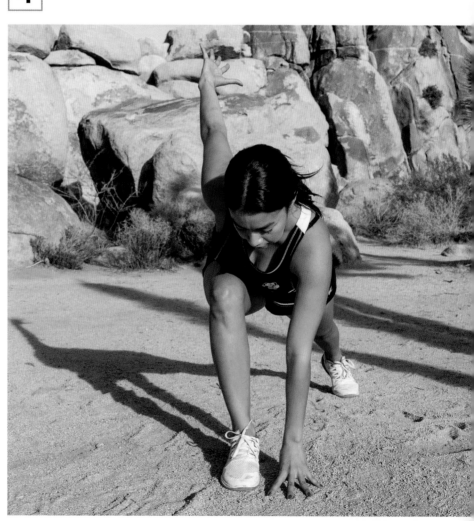

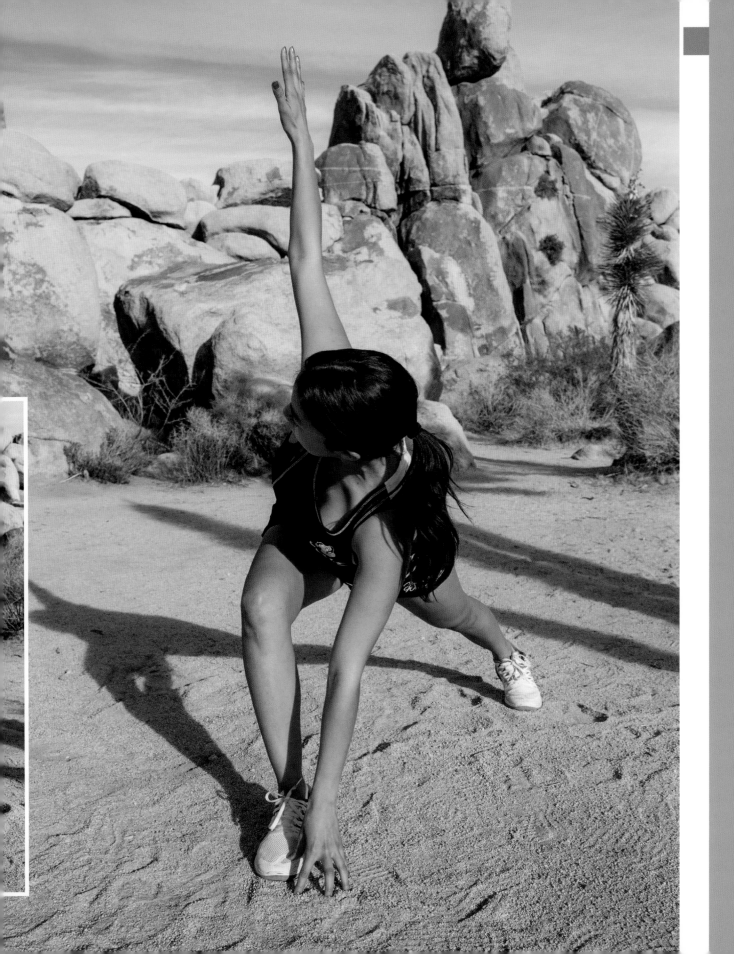

PRIMARY MUSCLE ACTION

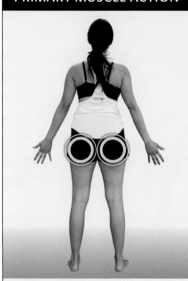

- Glutes
- Quadriceps
- Hamstrings
- Core
- Calves

DIAGONAL LUNGE

PROGRESSION

1 Begin in a standing position with your hands on your hips.

2 Take a big diagonal step outward with your left leg, rotating your right ankle in the same direction at the same time.

3 Bend both legs until your left thigh is parallel to the ground and your right knee is nearly touching the ground.

4 Push off the left heel to return to the starting position, and complete 12–15 repetitions, then switch to the opposite leg.

VARIATION

Try alternating legs for an increased challenge.

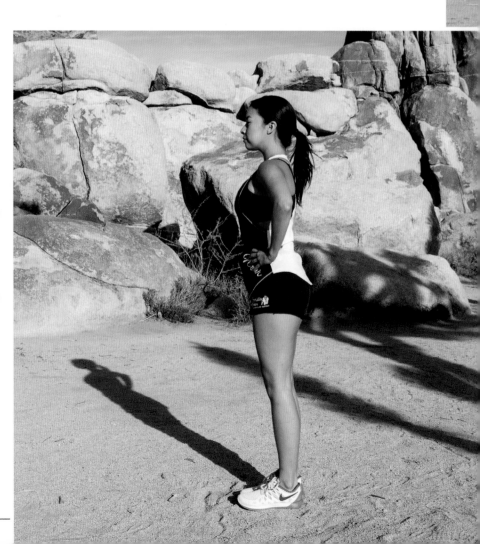

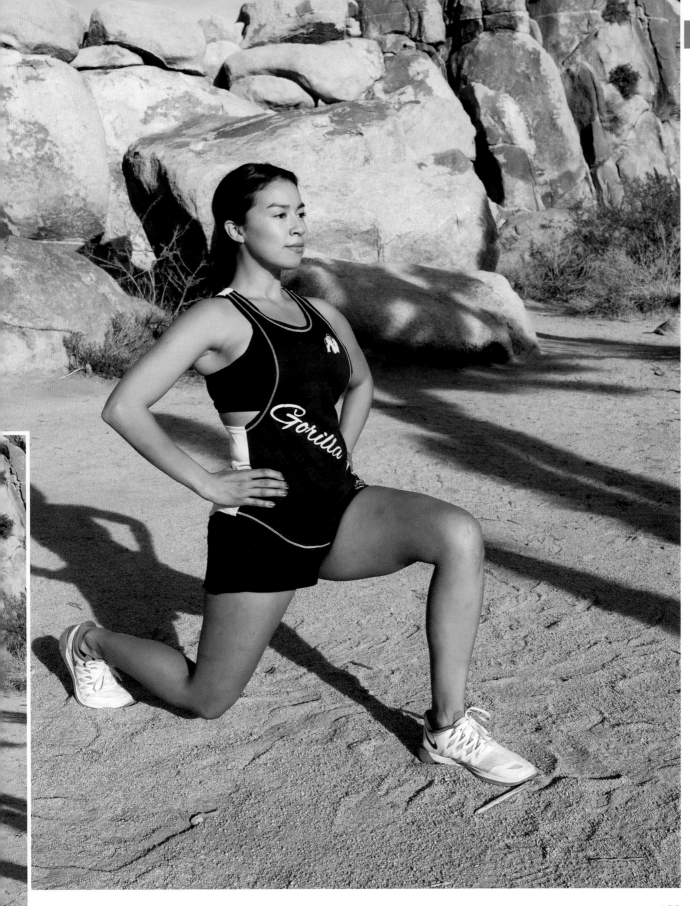

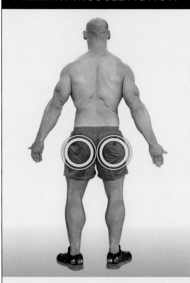

PRIMARY MUSCLE ACTION

- Glutes
- Quadriceps
- Hamstrings
- Core
- Calves
- Deltoids
- Triceps

SQUAT WITH TRANSVERSE PRESS

PROGRESSION

1 Begin in a standing position while holding a medicine ball in your left hand near your shoulder.

2 Squat downward while keeping your core tight and the medicine ball near your left shoulder.

3 As you ascend, simultaneously push the left arm up to full extension and rotate your torso to the right.

4 Lower yourself back down, and complete 12–15 repetitions, then switch to the right hand and left rotations for another 12–15 reps.

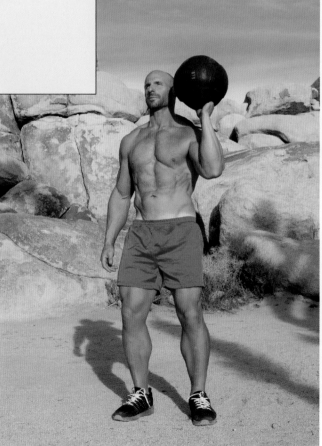

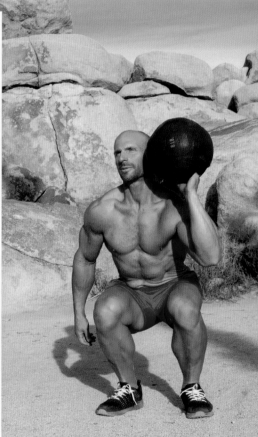

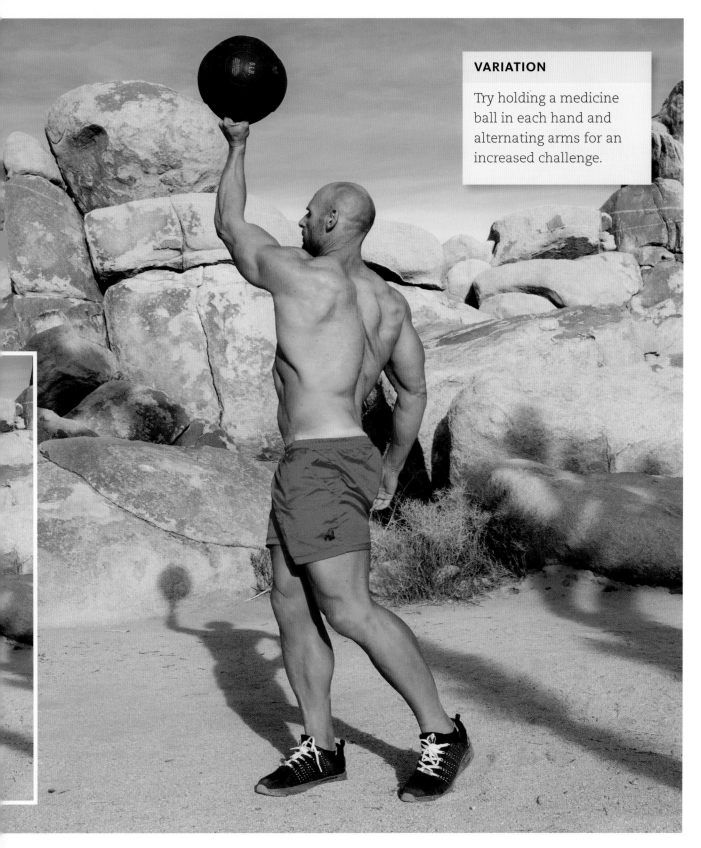

VARIATION

Try holding a medicine ball in each hand and alternating arms for an increased challenge.

PRIMARY MUSCLE ACTION

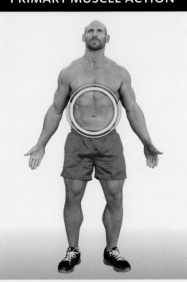

- Abdominals
- Obliques
- Intercostals

IRON CROSS

PROGRESSION

1 Lie on your back, with your legs straight up in the air and your arms out to the sides, palms downward.

2 Lower your legs to one side while keeping your torso stabilized and your back relatively braced against the ground.

3 Raise your legs back up to the starting point, and lower them to the opposite side, completing 15 repetitions per side.

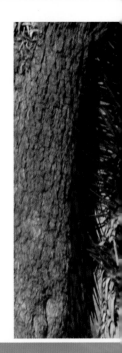

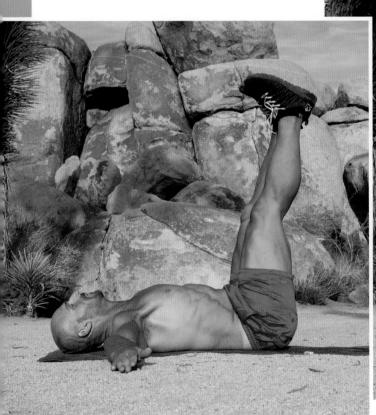

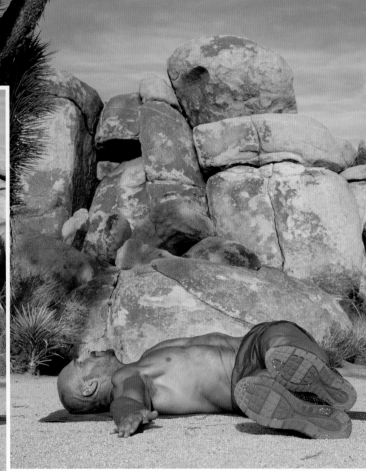

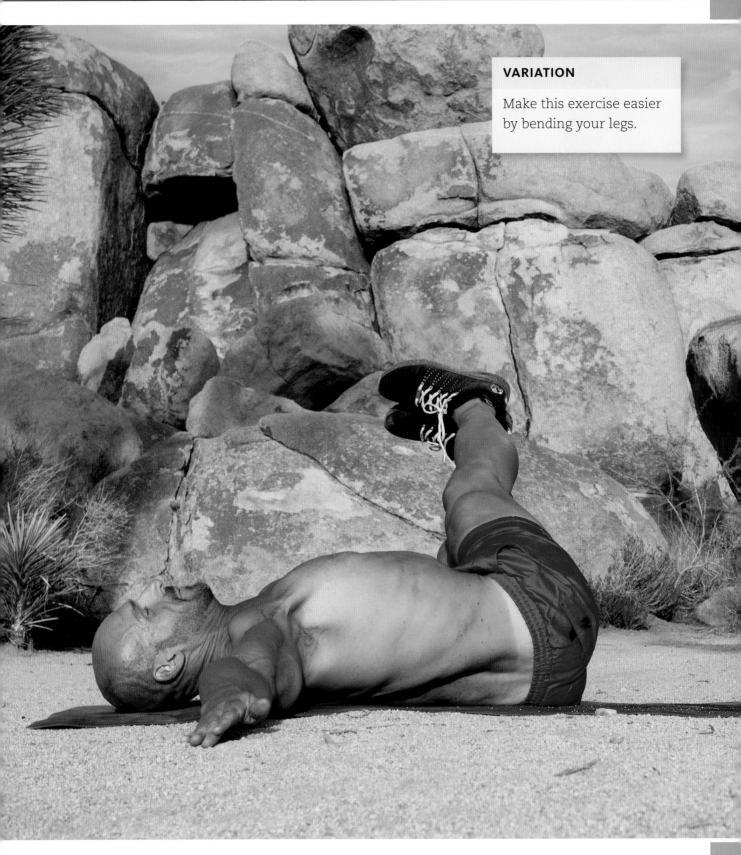

VARIATION

Make this exercise easier by bending your legs.

PRIMARY MUSCLE ACTION

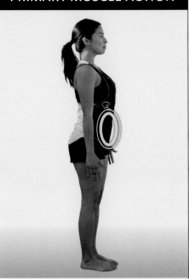

- Abdominals
- Obliques
- Intercostals

SIDE V-UP

PROGRESSION

1 Lie on your right side, with your right arm outstretched in front and your left hand on the back of your head, elbow facing upward.

2 Lift your legs while keeping them straight, and move your left elbow toward your knees.

3 Lower yourself back to the starting position without letting your feet touch the ground.

4 Complete 12–15 repetitions, then switch sides.

VARIATION

Try placing the stabilizing arm at your side for an increased challenge.

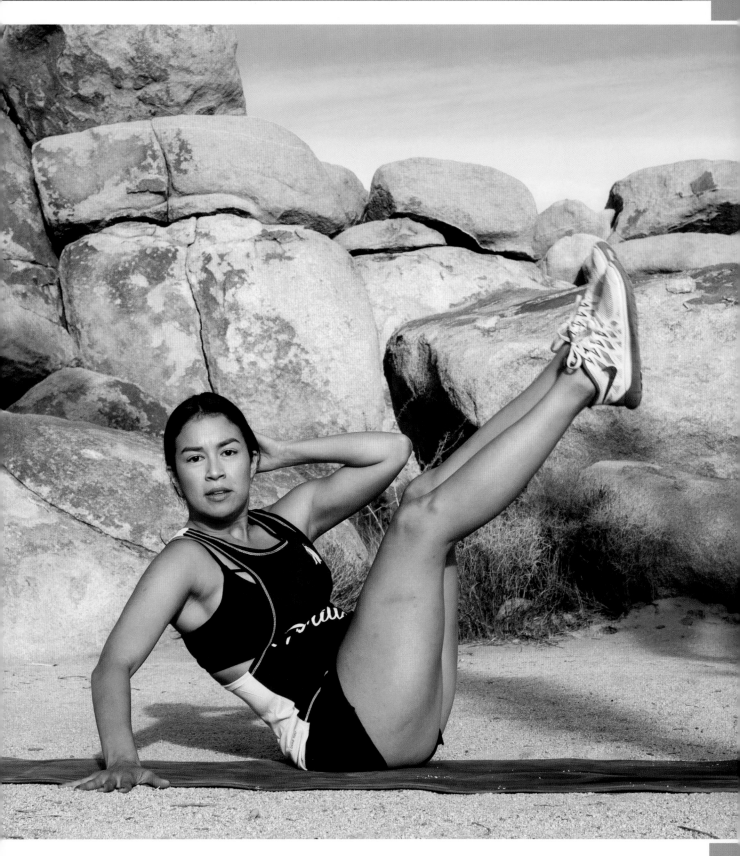

PRIMARY MUSCLE ACTION

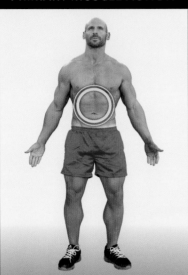

- Abdominals
- Obliques

RUSSIAN TWIST

PROGRESSION

1 In a seated position with your legs apart, hold a medicine ball in front of you with outstretched arms.

2 Lean back slightly while maintaining a flat back, and rotate your torso from one side to the other while keeping your arms up.

3 Complete 20 repetitions per side.

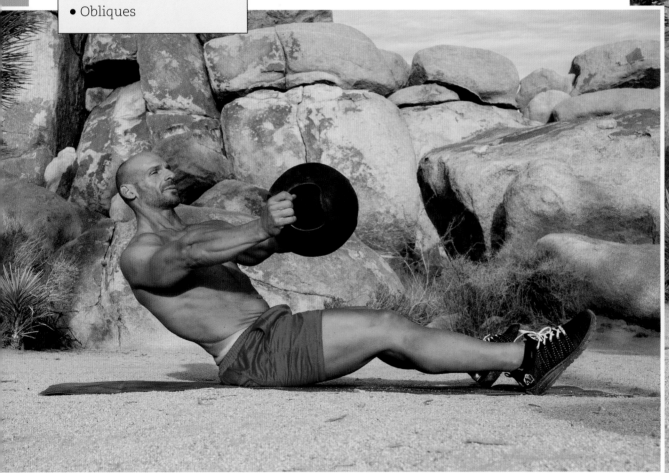

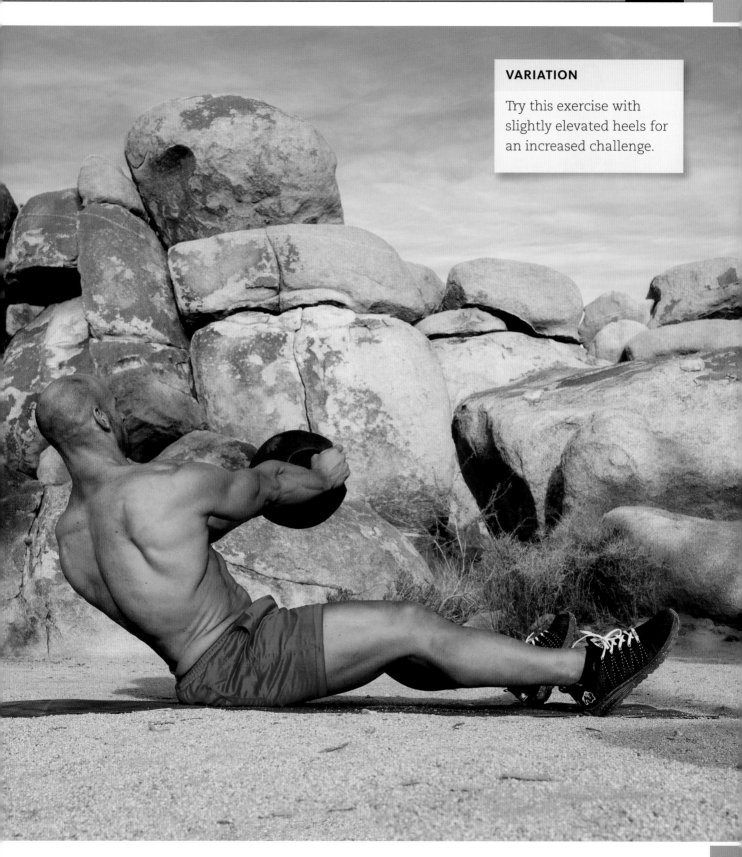

VARIATION

Try this exercise with slightly elevated heels for an increased challenge.

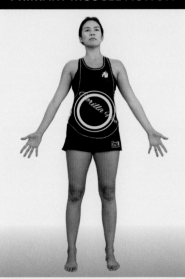

PRIMARY MUSCLE ACTION

- Abdominals
- Obliques
- Deltoids
- Lats

MEDICINE-BALL CHOP

PROGRESSION

1 In a standing position with feet just over shoulder-width apart, hold a medicine ball in front of your chest.

2 Rotate your torso to one side while extending your arms, also raising them slightly upward.

3 Quickly rotate back through the same pathway with extended arms, then continue on all the way through, while simultaneously extending and lowering your arms slightly downward.

4 Complete the full range of motion quickly for 15–20 repetitions, then switch sides.

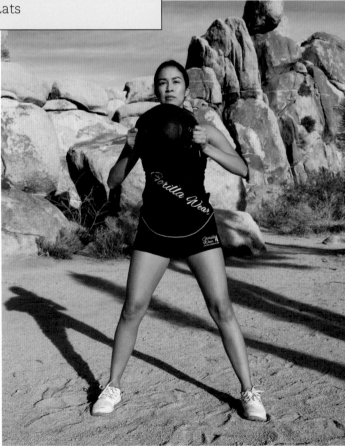

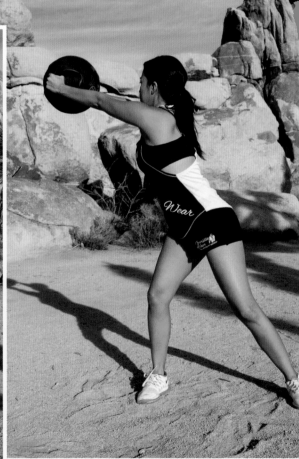

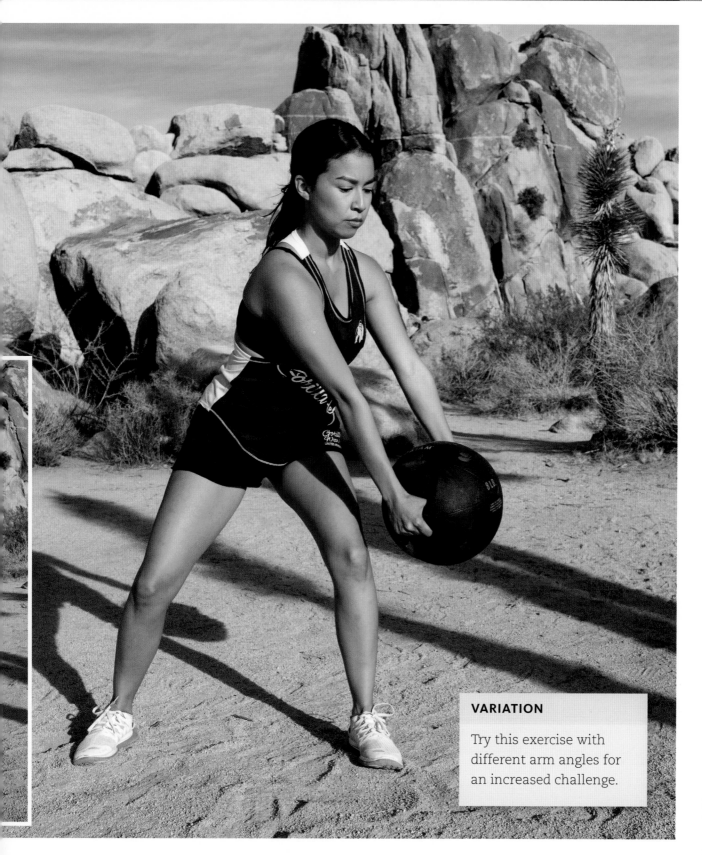

VARIATION

Try this exercise with different arm angles for an increased challenge.

PRIMARY MUSCLE ACTION

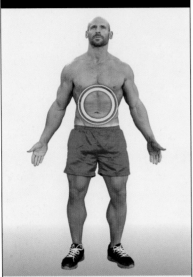

- Abdominals
- Obliques
- Deltoids
- Triceps

SIDE PLANK ROTATION

PROGRESSION

1 Begin in a traditional plank position.

2 Rotate your entire body to one side, while keeping one forearm planted and your core stabilized.

3 Return, complete 12–15 repetitions, then switch to the other side.

VARIATION

Try alternating sides for an increased challenge.

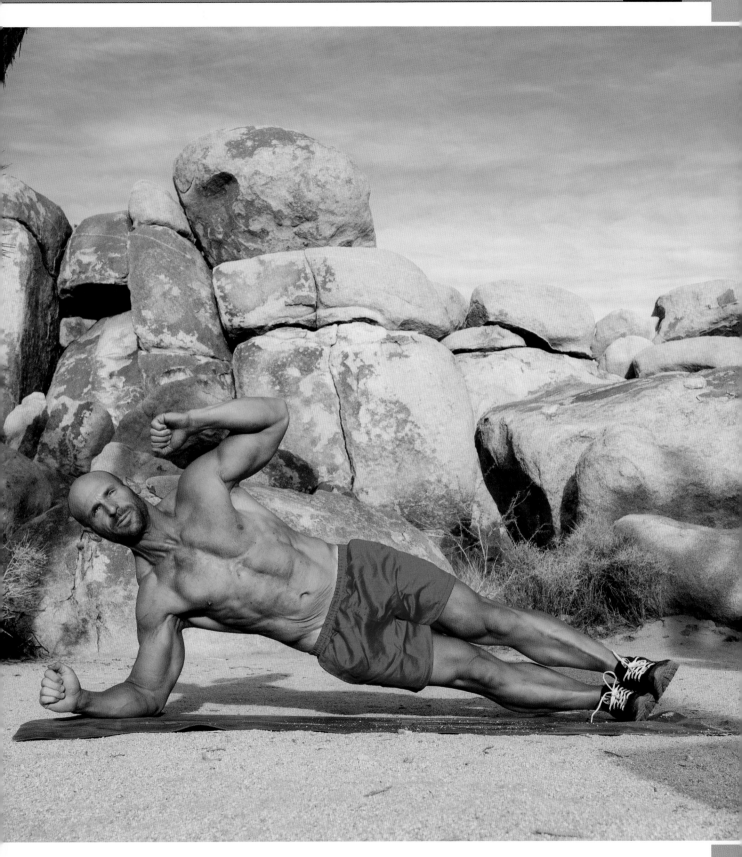

DIAGONAL CRUNCH WITH MEDICINE BALL

PRIMARY MUSCLE ACTION

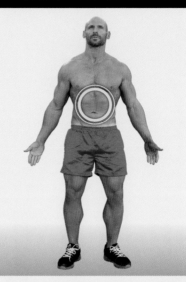

- Abdominals
- Obliques

PROGRESSION

1 Lie on your back with arms and legs outstretched, while holding a medicine ball in your hands.

2 Raise your arms and torso forward, then rotate your torso toward the right side.

3 Lower, return to the starting position, and alternate with your left side for 20 repetitions.

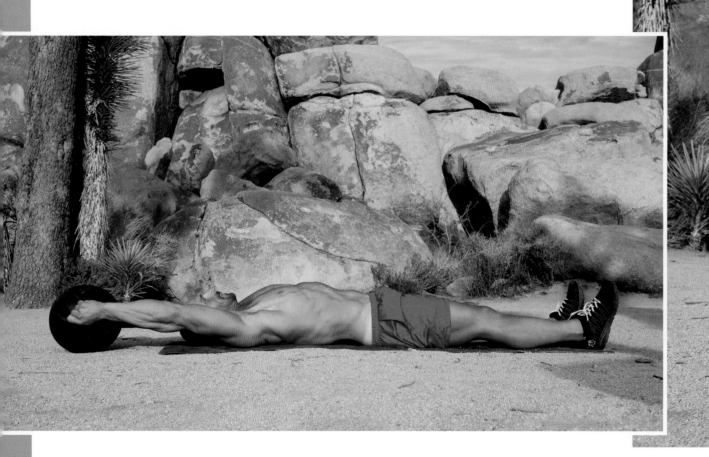

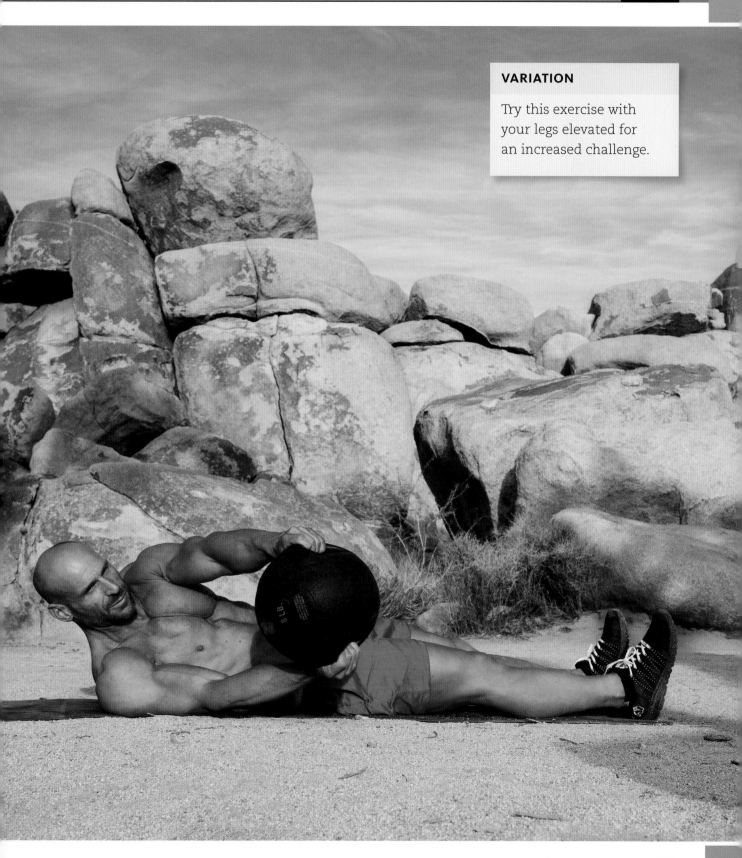

VARIATION

Try this exercise with your legs elevated for an increased challenge.

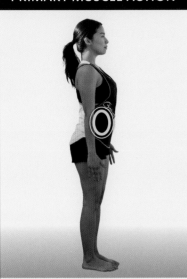

PRIMARY MUSCLE ACTION

- Obliques
- Core

HELICOPTER

PROGRESSION

1 Begin by standing with your arms at your sides.

2 Rotate your torso to one side while following suit with your head and raised arms.

3 Continue on to the other side until you have completed 50 repetitions per side.

VARIATION

Try this exercise while holding a medicine ball for an increased challenge.

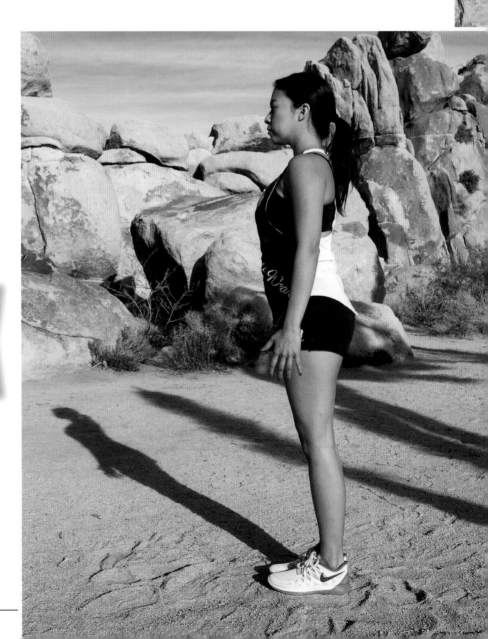

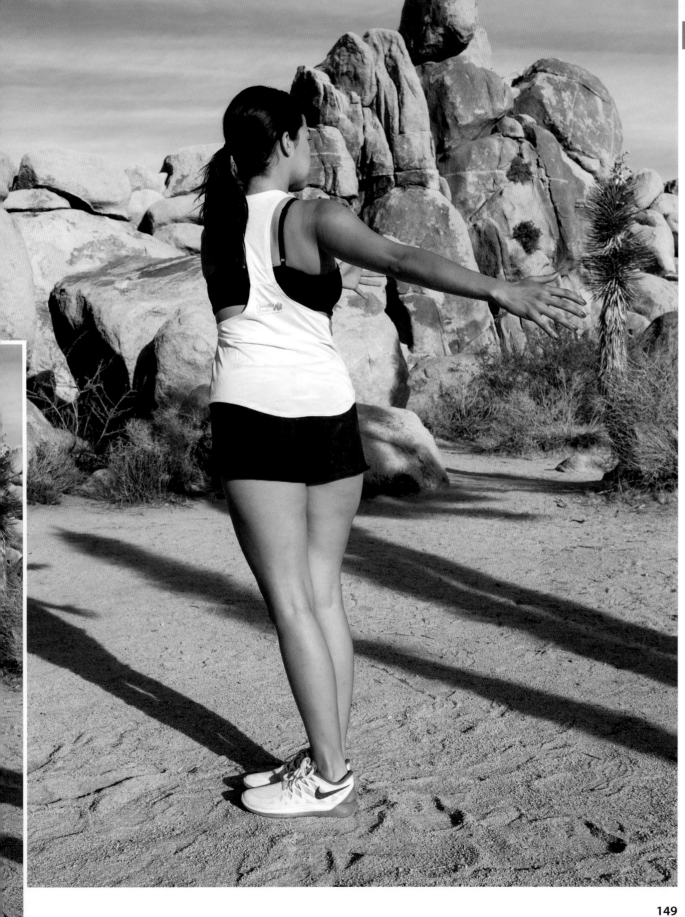

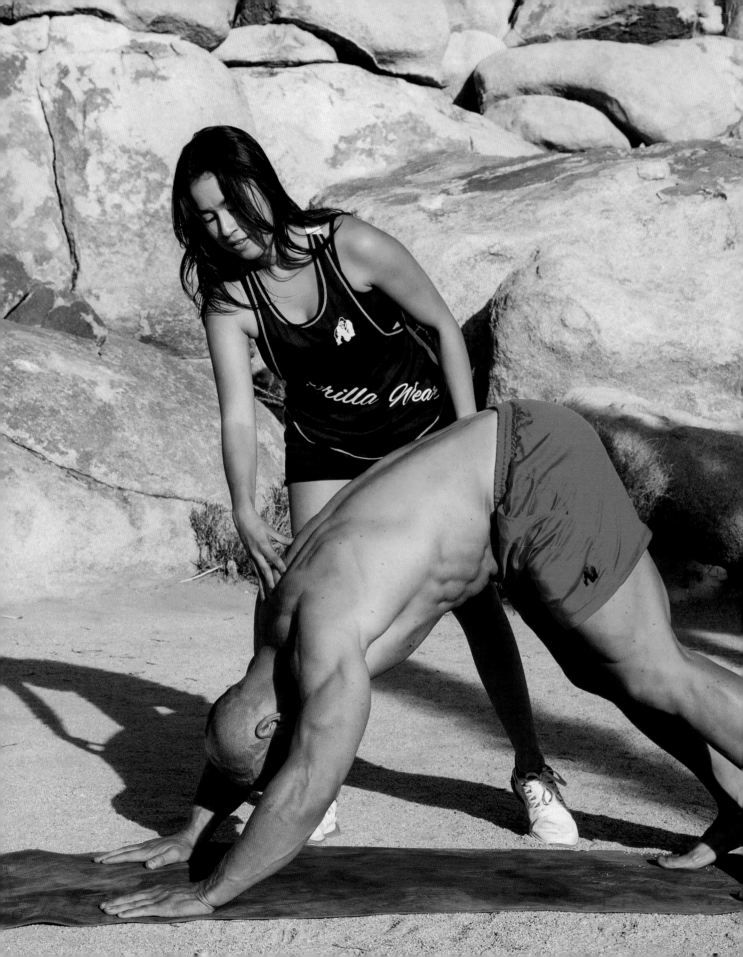

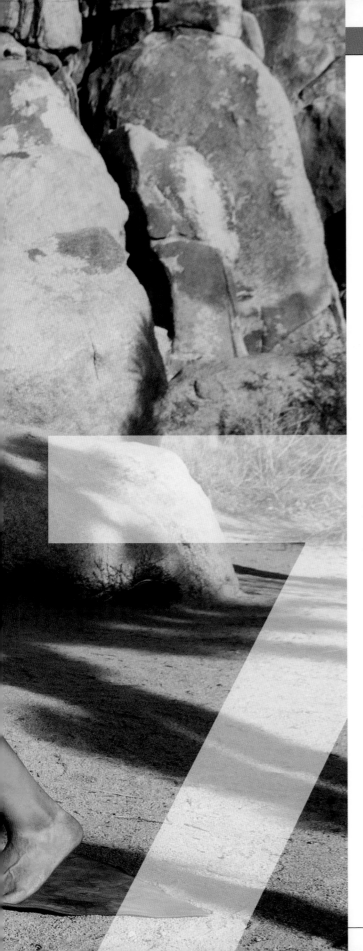

SPECIALTY MODALITIES

The exercises in this chapter are offered not as alternatives or substitutes but as an integral part of your arsenal. Of utmost concern is keeping yourself injury-free and functional. Progress can come in many forms and need not be measured by bigger arms or a more impressive bench press. In *Outdoor Physique*, we are striving for something more timeless and precious: the moving you.

In the old days, we might have ventured into a gym and raised a loaded barbell above our head at arms' length without so much as a warm-up. Or bounce rattling plates off our chest with a curved lower back to minimize the distance, and move a heavier given weight from point A to point B. As previously stated, as time goes on and the body matures, its abilities—and perhaps even its needs—change or diminish.

The moving you is about fortifying muscles—not for lifting maximal loads but simply for moving comfortably and with ease. The three specialty modalities included here—mobility movements, boxing, and yoga—are inserted both before and after your workouts to ensure you get a proper warm-up, unrestricted movement, and a cool-down.

Specifically, mobility movements help keep your body in the best shape it can be, regardless of age or ability. Although they might seem the least exciting part of your routine, their inclusion is a small price to pay for the gift of free and unrestricted movement.

MOBILITY MOVEMENTS help you move better by facilitating free motion around an uninhibited joint.

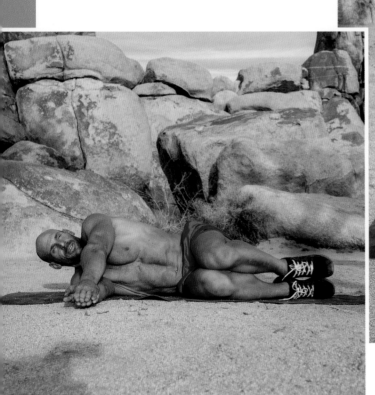

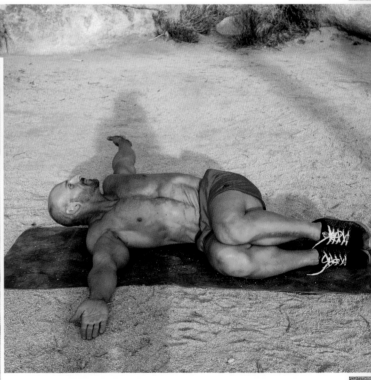

PRIMARY MUSCLE ACTION

- Deltoids
- Lats

CLAM-SHELL STRETCH

PROGRESSION

1 Lie on your right side with your legs bent, the left one on top of the right, and your arms stretched out in front of you with your hands together.

2 Raise the top arm and move it skyward. Keep moving it toward the other side, always following with your head.

3 Next, move the same arm above and past your head, again following it with your head. Continue the movement until you reach your starting position. Repeat 15 times, before switching to lie on your left side.

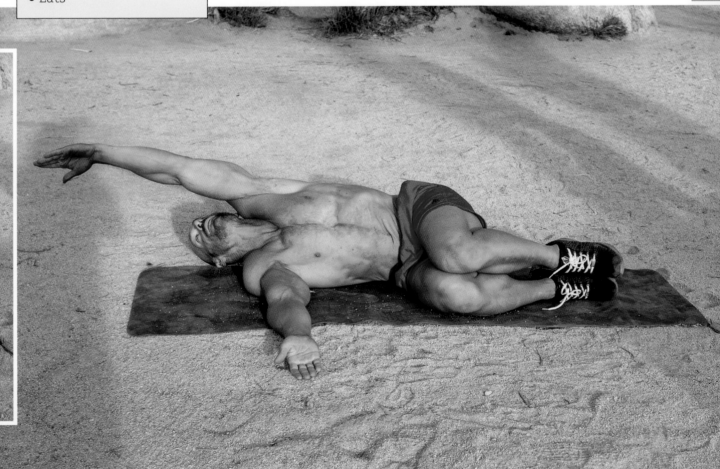

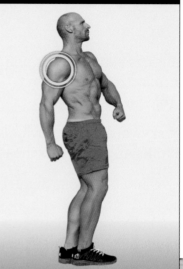

PRIMARY MUSCLE ACTION

- Deltoids

SHOULDER STRETCH

PROGRESSION

1 In a standing position, interlock your fingers behind you, palms down. While leaning forward, pull your arms up to fully engage the shoulders.

2 Hold for 30 seconds, release, and repeat three times.

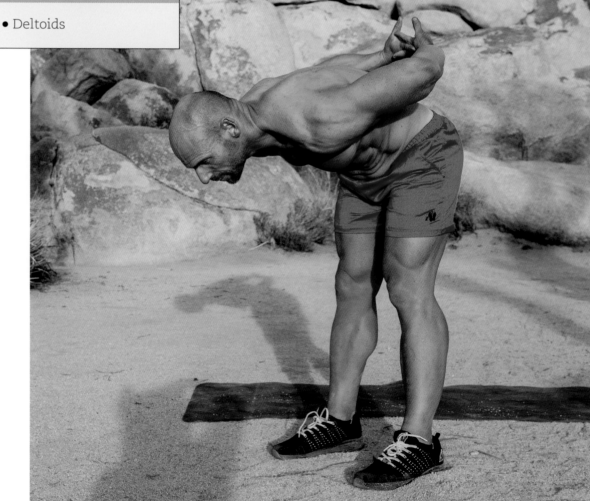

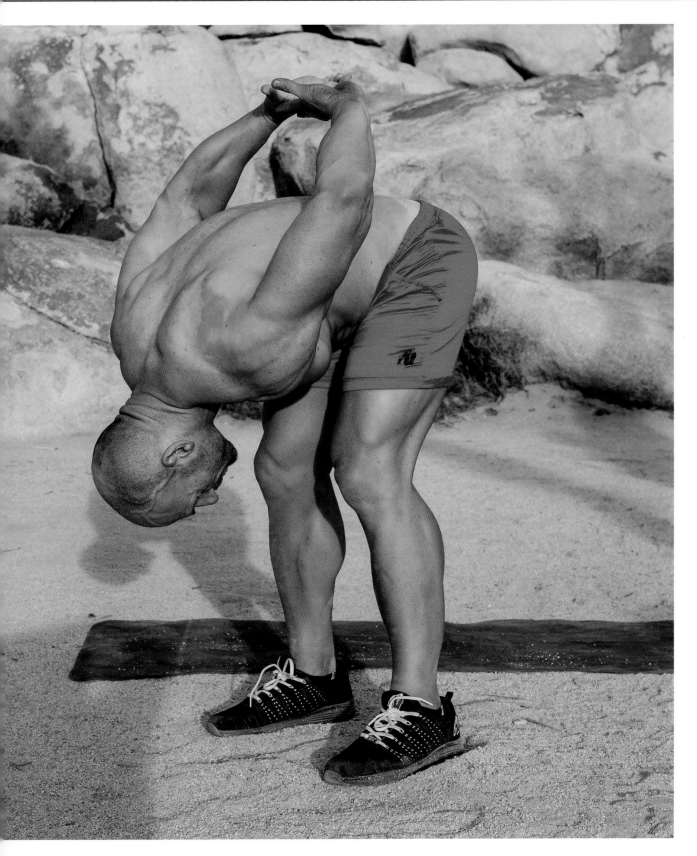

PRIMARY MUSCLE ACTION

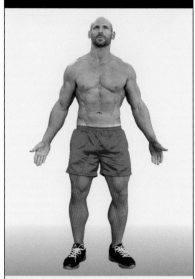

● Entire Body

STEP AND TWIST

PROGRESSION

1 Begin with your right leg bent in front, foot firmly planted, and your left leg stretched out behind you, balancing on its toes.

2 Place your left hand next to your right foot, and loop your right arm between your right leg and left arm.

3 Rotate your torso to the right as you raise your right arm high above you and turn your head to follow it, while also lowering your left knee to the ground. Return the arm and left knee, then repeat 15 times, before switching sides.

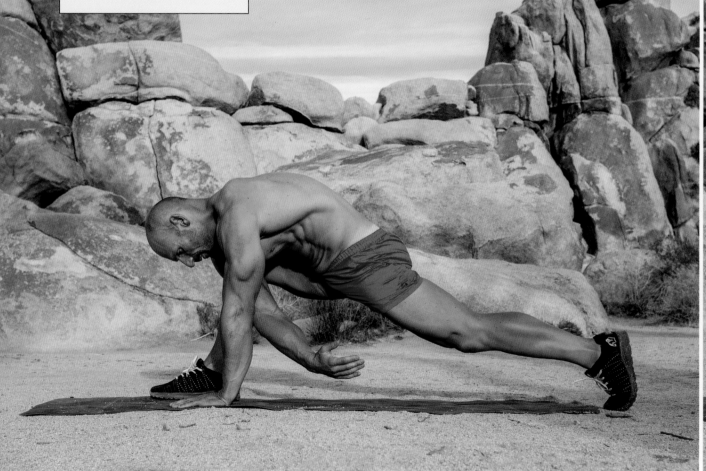

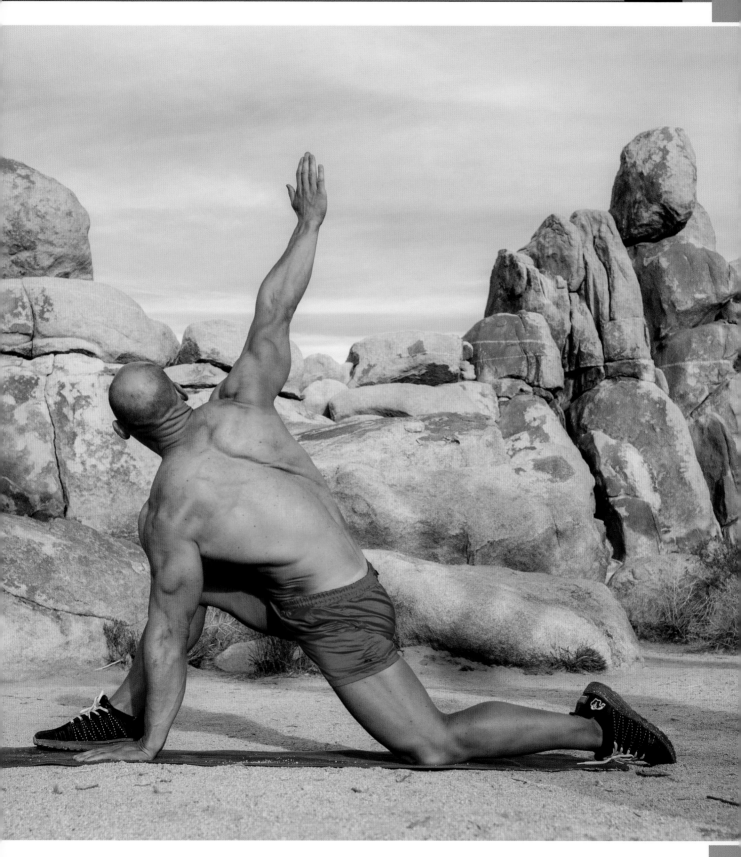

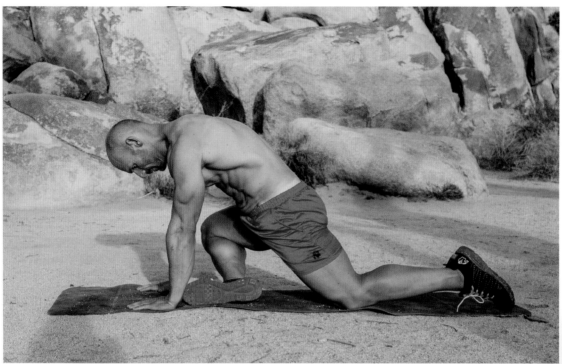

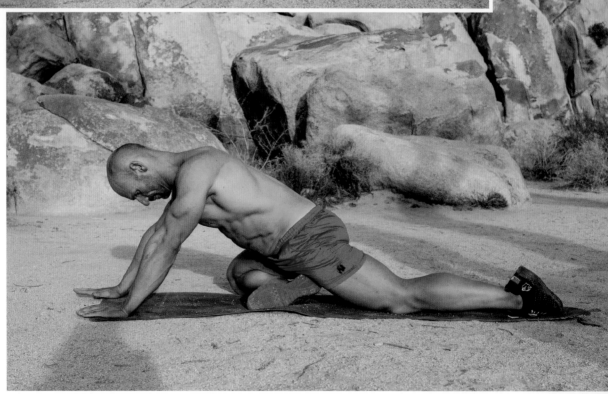

PIGEON POSE

PROGRESSION

1 Begin on your hands and knees. Bring your right knee toward your left hand and slide your left foot backward. Bring the right foot through toward the left hand, so that it is in line with the left leg.

2 Push backward, moving your pelvis closer to your right leg and continuing to lengthen the back leg.

3 Finally, bend your arms, leaning closer to the ground while also bringing your left leg toward the ground. Hold for 30–45 seconds, then repeat three times before moving on to the other leg.

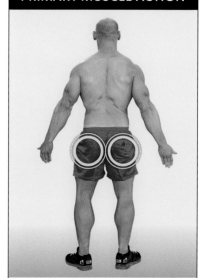

PRIMARY MUSCLE ACTION

- Hips
- Glutes

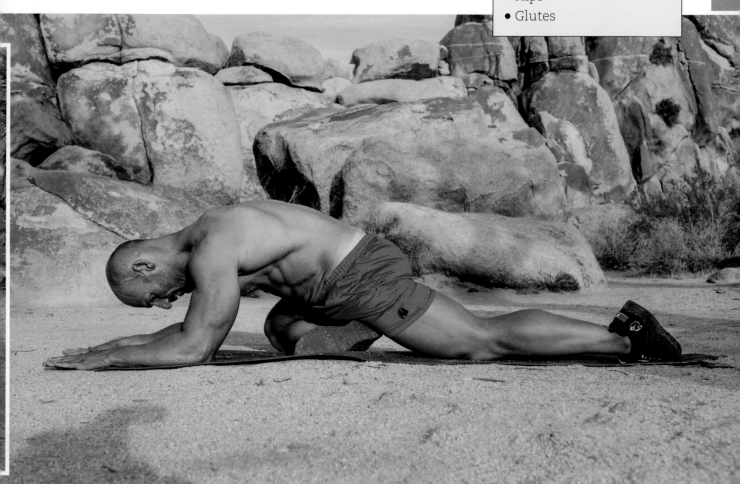

PRIMARY MUSCLE ACTION

• Hamstrings

ACTIVE HAMSTRING STRETCH

PROGRESSION

1 Begin by going down onto your right knee, with your right foot on its toes. Check that your left leg is at a 90-degree angle.

2 Place your fingertips on the ground, spread out, on either side of your left foot.

3 Raise your body up while keeping your fingertips on the ground, and straighten your back leg, feeling an intense stretch in your hamstrings.

4 Hold for 15–30 seconds, then repeat three times before moving on to the other leg.

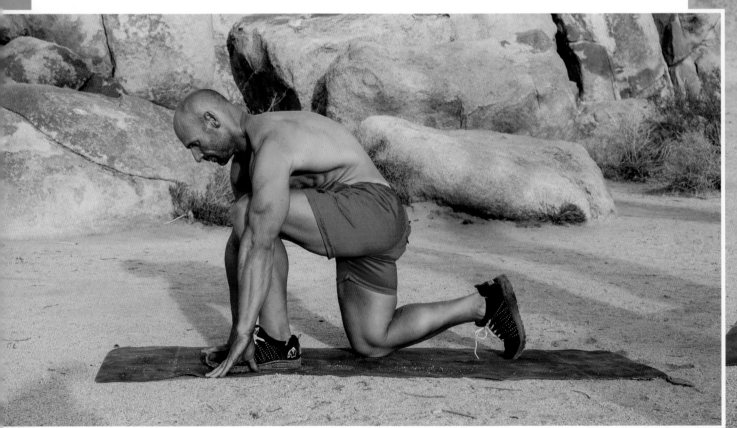

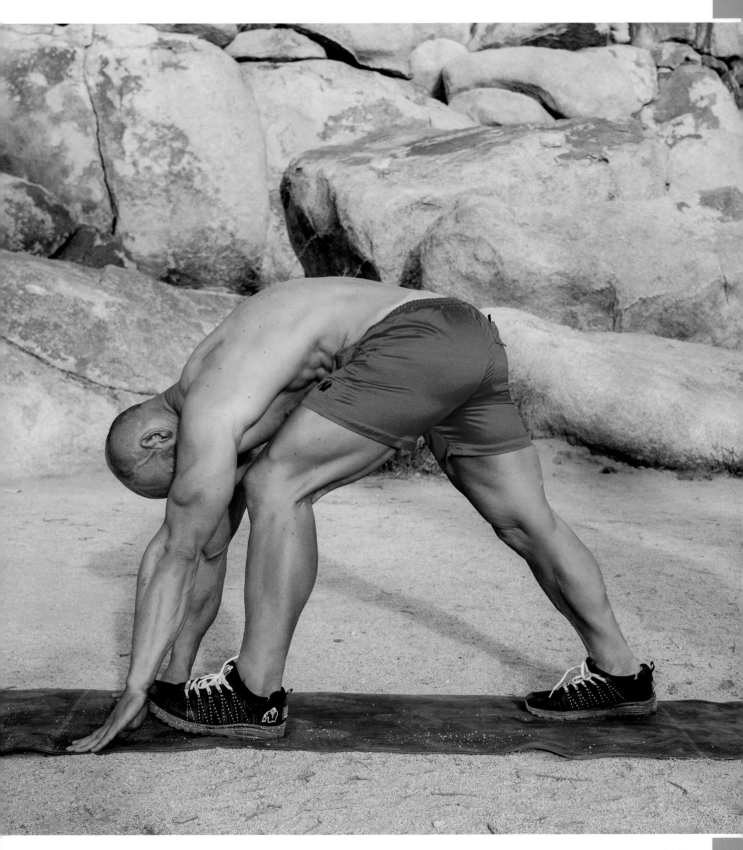

BOXING combinations are included in this book to help make cardio more fun, as well as to offer a reprieve from the traditional and often redundant tedium of steadfast, predictable cardiovascular movement patterns.

FIGHTER'S STANCE

PROGRESSION

1 Begin in a standing position with your feet apart and your knees slightly bent.

2 Angle your torso and body diagonally toward your "opponent," as opposed to straight on, so that your left foot is slightly forward.

3 Keeping your chin down, your head up, and your elbows in, raise your right fist toward the right side of your face and the left fist in front of it.

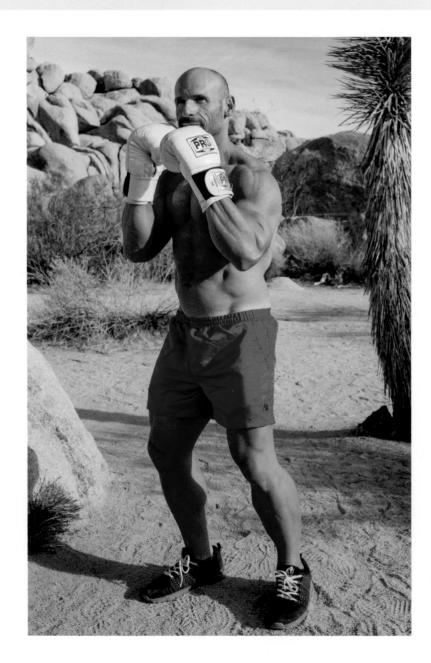

PRIMARY MUSCLE ACTION

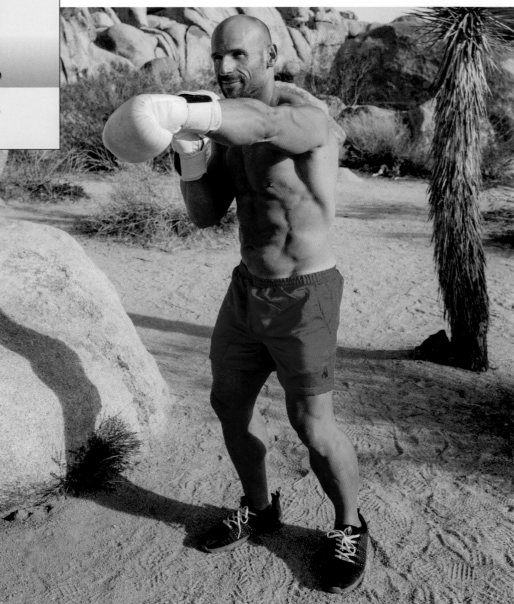

- Anterior Deltoids
- Pectorals

JAB
PROGRESSION

1 While in the fighter's stance, with your left hand in front of your face, extend your fist toward your opponent as you exhale.

2 For more power, rotate your arm inward as you throw the punch, so your fist finishes palm down.

PRIMARY MUSCLE ACTION

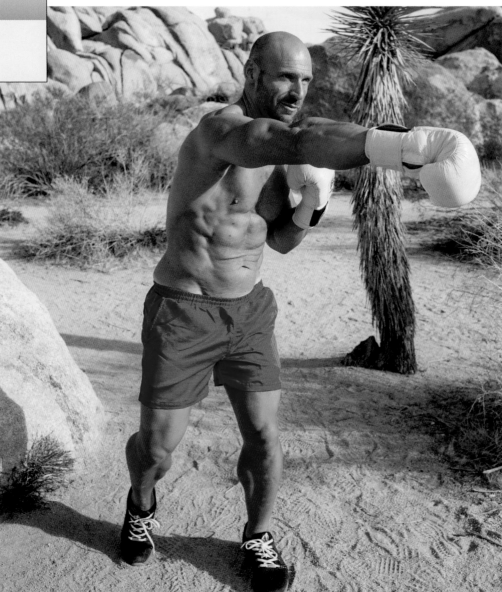

- Core
- Deltoids

CROSS

PROGRESSION

1 While in the fighter's stance, keep your front foot flat on the ground and your rear foot up on your toes.

2 As you throw your cocked hand (the opposite hand to the front foot) directly from the chin and toward your opponent, palm down, rotate the rear foot, knee, and hip inward to deliver more power.

3 Pull back your left shoulder to counterbalance after the punch is delivered.

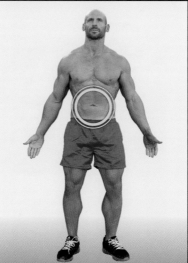

• Core

HOOK

PROGRESSION

1 From the fighter's stance, with the left hand in front of your face, move your left hand downward, so that it is parallel to the floor.

2 Rotate your core and your back inward in a horizontal arc toward your opponent's midriff as you throw the punch with your left arm.

3 Be sure to rotate the body and pivot your lead foot for maximum power.

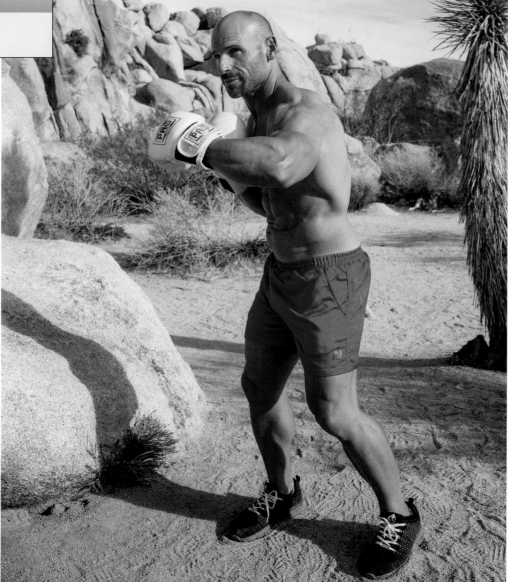

UPPERCUT

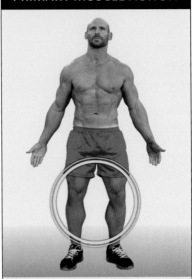

PRIMARY MUSCLE ACTION

- Legs
- Core
- Shoulders

PROGRESSION

1 While in the fighter's stance, plant your left foot flat on the ground and bring your right foot up onto its toes.

2 As you throw your cocked right hand directly from the chin and at an upward angle, rotate the right foot, knee, and hip inward to deliver more power.

3 Pull the fist straight back to your chin once the punch has been delivered.

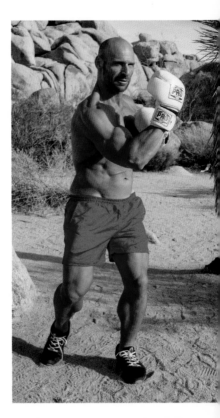

DUCK

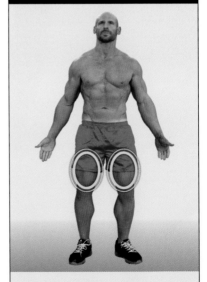

PRIMARY MUSCLE ACTION

- Quadriceps

PROGRESSION

1 The duck is a defensive measure that can quickly become an offensive maneuver by throwing your own punches. Begin in the squared-up fighter's stance, with your back straight.

2 Keep your guard up at all times as you quickly bend the knees and drop low enough to avoid your opponent's offense.

3 Be sure to keep your eyes up at all times, and rise up ready to counter as you quickly return to the starting position.

BOXING SEQUENCES

The boxing sequences implemented in your workouts are as follows:

PHASE 1:
1. jab
2. jab, cross
3. jab, jab, cross
4. jab, jab, cross, hook
5. jab, jab, cross, hook, duck
6. jab, jab, cross, hook, duck, uppercut
6. jab, jab, cross, hook, duck, uppercut
5. jab, jab, cross, hook, duck
4. jab, jab, cross, hook
3. jab, jab, cross
2. jab, cross
1. jab

PHASE 2:
1. jab
2. jab, cross
3. jab, jab, cross
4. jab, jab, cross, hook
5. jab, jab, cross, hook, duck
6. jab, jab, cross, hook, duck, uppercut
7. jab, jab, cross, hook, duck, uppercut, jab
8. jab, jab, cross, hook, duck, uppercut, jab, uppercut
9. jab, jab, cross, hook, duck, uppercut, jab, uppercut, duck
9. jab, jab, cross, hook, duck, uppercut, jab, uppercut, duck
8. jab, jab, cross, hook, duck, uppercut, jab, uppercut
7. jab, jab, cross, hook, duck, uppercut, jab
6. jab, jab, cross, hook, duck, uppercut
5. jab, jab, cross, hook, duck
4. jab, jab, cross, hook
3. jab, jab, cross
2. jab, cross
1. jab

PHASE 3:
1. jab
2. jab, cross
3. jab, jab, cross
4. jab, jab, cross, hook
5. jab, jab, cross, hook, duck
6. jab, jab, cross, hook, duck, uppercut
7. jab, jab, cross, hook, duck, uppercut, jab
8. jab, jab, cross, hook, duck, uppercut, jab, uppercut
9. jab, jab, cross, hook, duck, uppercut, jab, uppercut, duck
10. jab, jab, cross, hook, duck, uppercut, jab, uppercut, duck, jab
11. jab, jab, cross, hook, duck, uppercut, jab, uppercut, duck, jab, cross
12. jab, jab, cross, hook, duck, uppercut, jab, uppercut, duck, jab, cross, jab
12. jab, jab, cross, hook, duck, uppercut, jab, uppercut, duck, jab, cross, jab
11. jab, jab, cross, hook, duck, uppercut, jab, uppercut, duck, jab, cross
10. jab, jab, cross, hook, duck, uppercut, jab, uppercut, duck, jab
9. jab, jab, cross, hook, duck, uppercut, jab, uppercut, duck
8. jab, jab, cross, hook, duck, uppercut, jab, uppercut
7. jab, jab, cross, hook, duck, uppercut, jab
6. jab, jab, cross, hook, duck, uppercut
5. jab, jab, cross, hook, duck
4. jab, jab, cross, hook
3. jab, jab, cross
2. jab, cross
1. jab

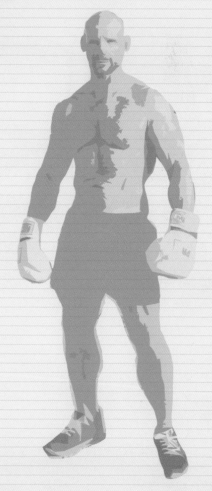

YOGA—an ancient Hindu series of disciplines—is included here as both an active-rest measure and a cool-down after your workouts. Its benefits are manifold, and it could be argued that yoga is the most organic form of bodyweight training.

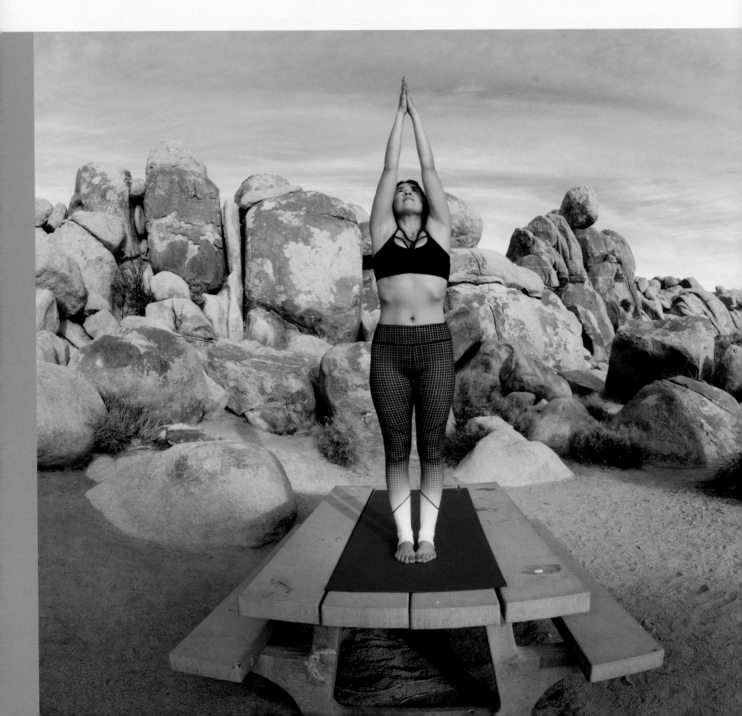

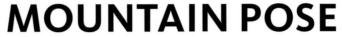

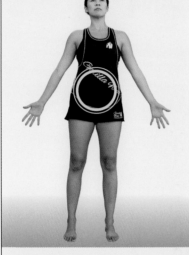

- Abdomen
- Glutes
- Quadriceps

MOUNTAIN POSE
TADASANA

PROGRESSION

1 Stand with your big toes touching. Spread and plant your toes softly on the ground, with your weight balanced evenly on your feet.

2 Hold your core in while lifting your chest and keeping your shoulders down.

3 Keep your palms facing inward while feeling your shoulder blades coming together. Hold for 5–8 breaths.

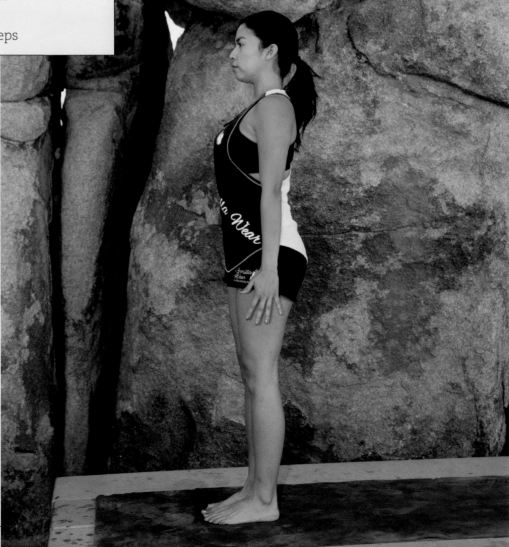

PRIMARY MUSCLE ACTION

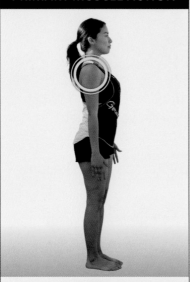

- Deltoids
- Hamstrings
- Calves
- Core
- Hips

DOWNWARD DOG
ADHO MUKHA SVANASANA

PROGRESSION

1 Get down on all fours, with your wrists under your shoulders and your knees under your hips. Raise your knees as your push your hips back toward your heels.

2 Straighten your legs if able while you carefully walk your hands forward.

3 Press through your palms while rotating your elbows toward one another. Be sure to keep your core and legs engaged. Hold for 5–8 breaths.

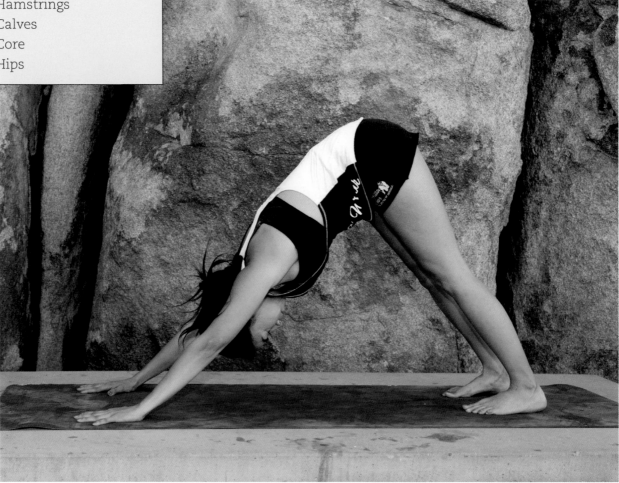

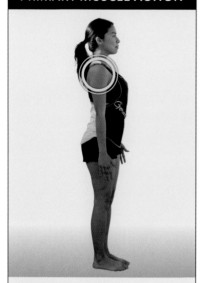

- Deltoids
- Hamstrings
- Calves
- Core
- Hips

THREE-LEGGED DOWNWARD DOG
EKA PADA ADHO MUKHA SVANASANA

PROGRESSION

1 Get down on all fours, with your wrists under your shoulders and your knees under your hips. Raise your knees as your push your hips back toward your heels.

2 Straighten your legs if able while you carefully walk your hands forward.

3 Press through your palms while rotating your elbows toward one another. Be sure to keep your core and legs engaged.

4 Lift one leg straight back and up in the air. Hold this position for 8–10 breaths, then switch legs.

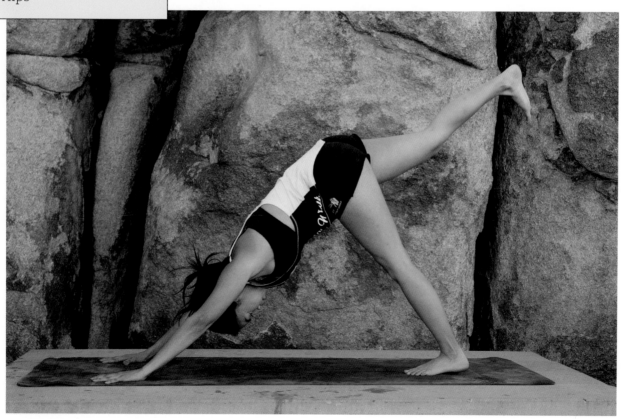

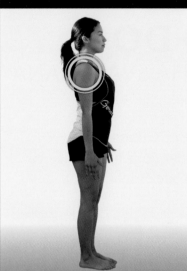

- Deltoids
- Arms
- Back
- Quadriceps
- Calves
- Pectorals

WARRIOR 1
VIRABHADRASANA I

PROGRESSION

1 Take a giant step back with your left foot, and sink into a soft lunge. Press your left heel down, then angle your left foot to 75 degrees.

2 Step forward slightly with the right foot, keeping your chest up. Raise your hands overhead, and press your palms together.

3 Hold for 8–10 breaths, then repeat on the other side.

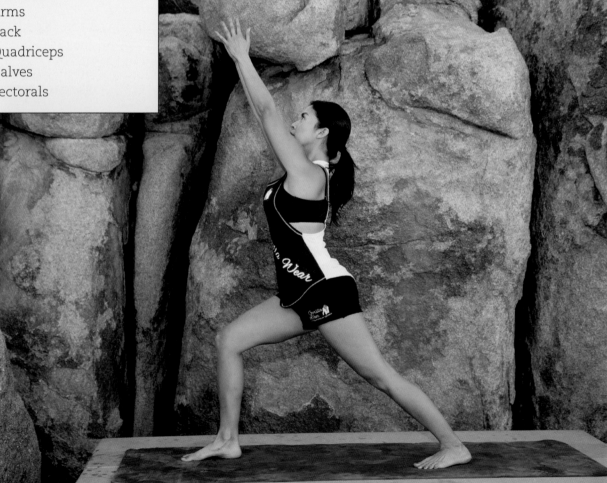

PRIMARY MUSCLE ACTION

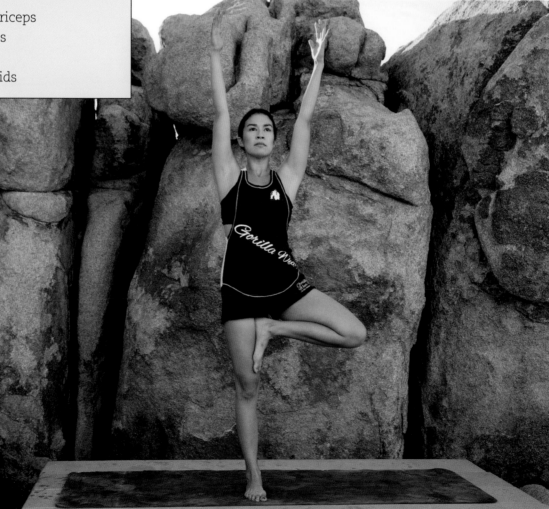

- Quadriceps
- Calves
- Core
- Deltoids

TREE POSE
VRKSASANA

PROGRESSION

1 Start in a standing position with your arms by your sides. Place the sole of one foot against the inner thigh of the other leg, with toes pointing down.

2 Raise your arms overhead with your fingers spread and palms facing one another.

3 Hold for 8–10 breaths, then return to the starting position before switching sides.

PRIMARY MUSCLE ACTION

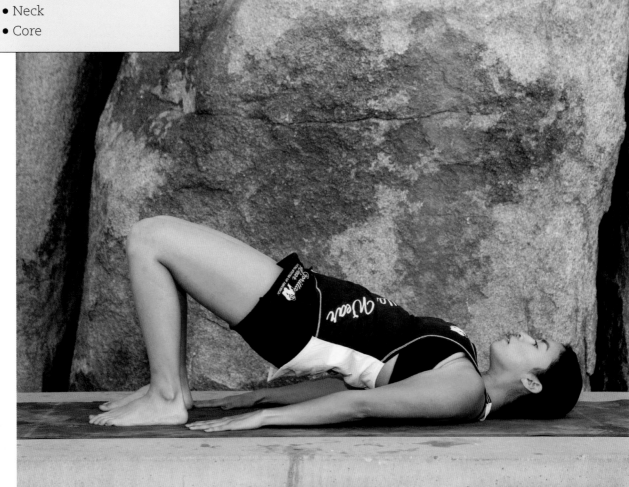

- Pectorals
- Neck
- Core

BRIDGE POSE
SETU BANDHA SARVANGASANA

PROGRESSION

1 Lie on your back with your knees raised, your feet planted hip-width apart, and your arms lengthened at your sides.

2 Push through your feet as you lift your rear off the ground, keeping your arms lengthened.

3 Hold for 8–10 breaths before returning to the starting position.

PRIMARY MUSCLE ACTION

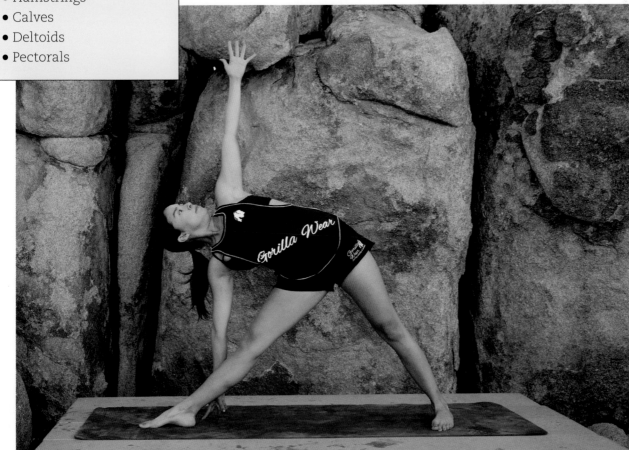

- Quadriceps
- Hips
- Hamstrings
- Calves
- Deltoids
- Pectorals

TRIANGLE POSE
TRIKONASANA

PROGRESSION

1 Stand with your feet wide apart, then raise both arms out to your sides, parallel to the ground.

2 Turn the right foot out by 90 degrees and the left by about 45 degrees.

3 Keep your core and quadriceps engaged as you hinge over to the right side while placing the fingertips of your right hand on or near the ground.

4 Look skyward, toward your left hand, and hold for 5–8 breaths. Return to the starting position, before repeating on the other side.

PRIMARY MUSCLE ACTION

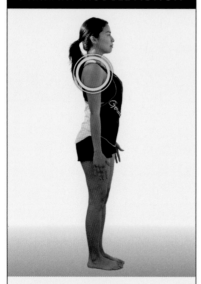

- Deltoids
- Hips
- Neck

HALF LORD OF THE FISHES POSE
ARDHA MATSYENDRASANA

PROGRESSION

1 Sit on the ground with straight legs, then bend your knees and slide your right foot under your left leg, so that your right foot is just on the outside of your left. Then step over the right leg with the left foot, allowing the left knee to point toward the sky.

2 Twist your torso toward the left as you press your left fingertips on the ground and your bent right arm on the outside of your left thigh, just above the knee.

3 Push the left foot into the ground, lengthen the torso and hold for 5–8 breaths. Repeat for the other side.

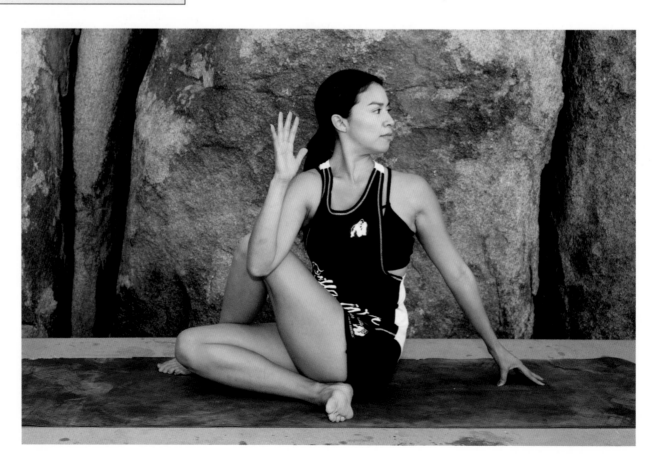

PRIMARY MUSCLE ACTION

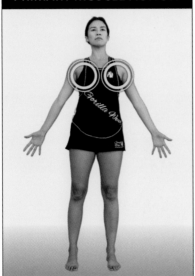

- Pectorals
- Deltoids
- Core

COBRA POSE
BHUJANGASANA

PROGRESSION

1 Lie face down with your legs stretched behind you and the tops of your feet facing downward. Spread your hands on the ground under your shoulders.

2 Push through your hands as you begin to straighten your arms but keeping them bent, and lift your chest up until you feel a connection throughout.

3 Hold for 8–10 breaths before returning to the starting position.

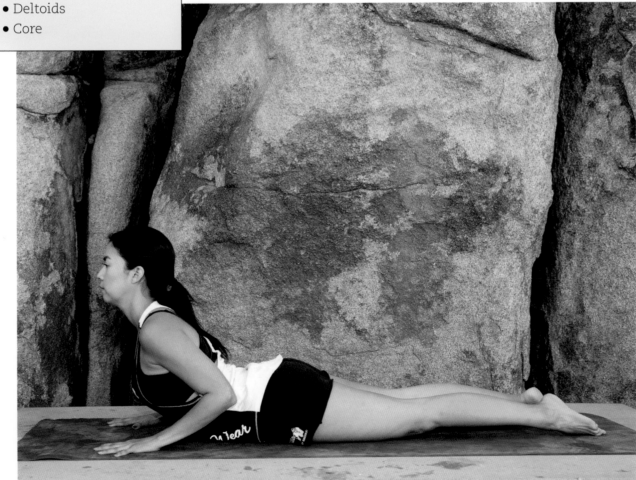

PRIMARY MUSCLE ACTION

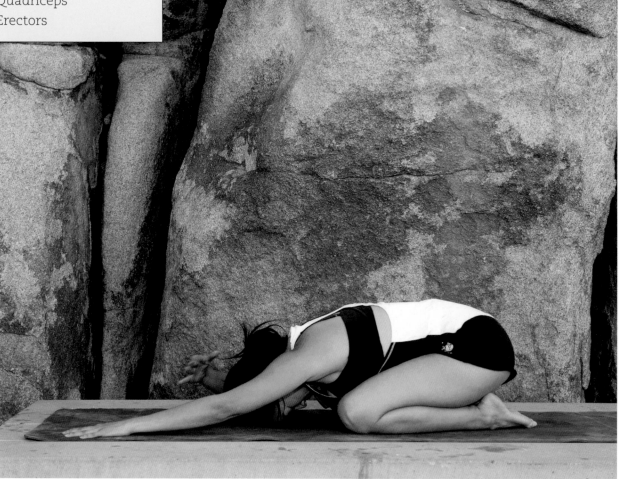

- Hips
- Quadriceps
- Erectors

CHILD'S POSE
BALASANA

PROGRESSION

1 Start on all fours, then bring your knees and feet together as you move your rear back toward your heels. At the same time, stretch your arms forward.

2 Lower your forehead to the ground, and let your body relax, releasing any tension.

3 Hold for 8–10 breaths.

FORWARD FOLD
UTTANASANA

PROGRESSION

1 From a standing position with your feet together, bend forward while keeping your legs soft but nearly locked. Let your arms reach downward, with your fingers spread. Place your palms on the ground if you are able.

2 Let your head hang, holding for 8–10 breaths, before slowly returning to the starting position.

PRIMARY MUSCLE ACTION

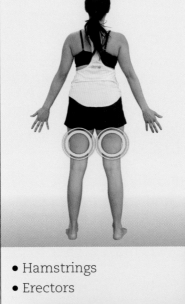

- Hamstrings
- Erectors

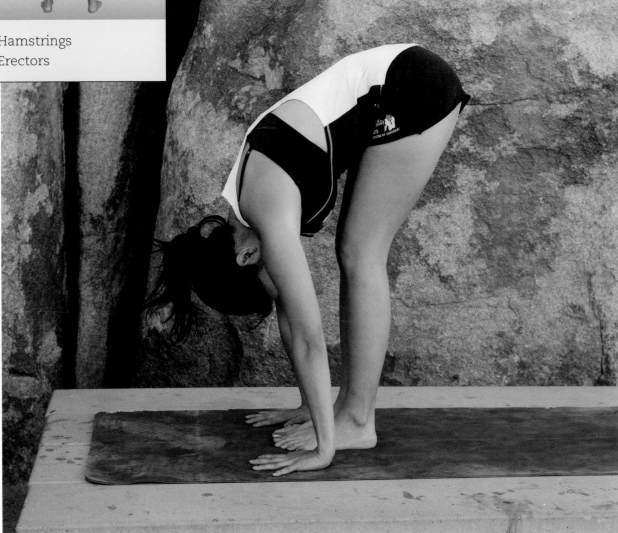

PRIMARY MUSCLE ACTION

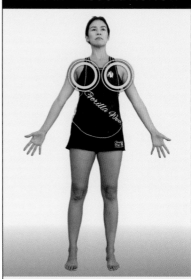

- Pectorals
- Deltoids
- Erectors

UPWARD-FACING DOG
URDHVA MUKHA SVANASANA

PROGRESSION

1 Lie face-down with your legs stretched behind you and the tops of your feet facing downward. Spread your hands on the ground under your shoulders.

2 Push through your hands as you fully straighten your arms and raise your torso and legs a few inches from the ground.

3 Hold for 8–10 breaths, before slowly moving back to the starting position.

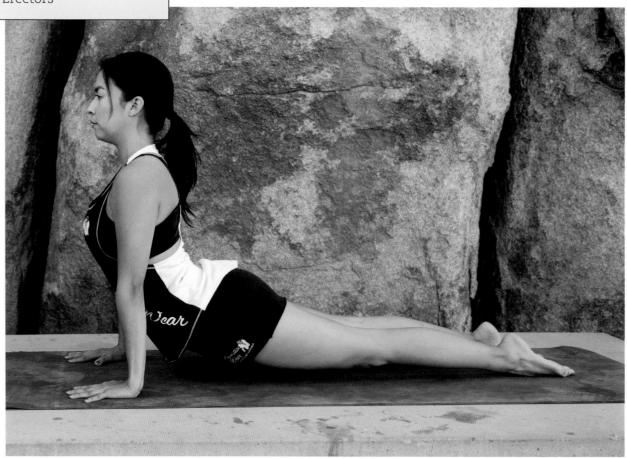

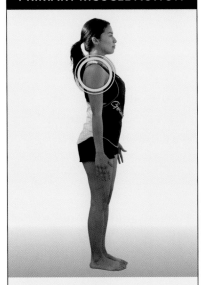

- Shoulders
- Hamstrings
- Calves
- Ankles
- Back

WARRIOR 3
VIRABHADRASANA III

PROGRESSION

1 Starting from a standing position with your hands at your sides, keep the right leg slightly bent as you lean forward through the torso while raising the left leg back and upward.

2 Raise your arms parallel to the ground and allow your head to drop, so that your arms, torso, and raised leg become one straight line.

3 Hold for 8–10 breaths before returning to the starting position and switching sides.

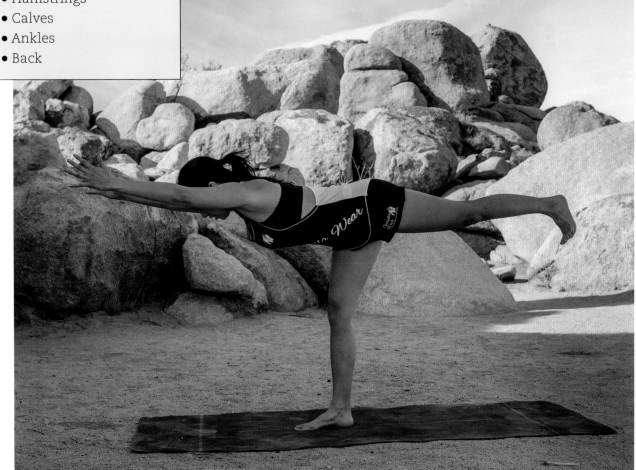

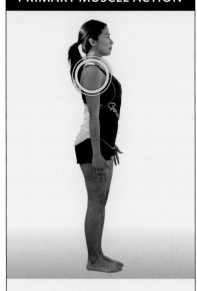

PRIMARY MUSCLE ACTION

- Deltoids
- Core

UPWARD SALUTE
URDHVA HASTASANA

PROGRESSION

1 Stand with your hands at your sides and your feet together, spread and planted softly on the ground, with your weight balanced evenly between them.

2 Keep your core in and your shoulders down while you lift your chest.

3 Turn your hands outward, and sweep your arms out to the sides and up toward the sky.

4 Press your palms and fingers together, and hold for 5–8 breaths.

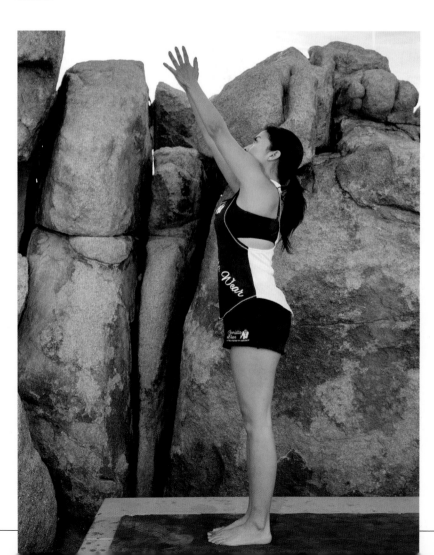

PRIMARY MUSCLE ACTION

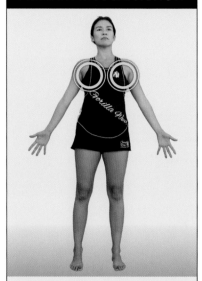

- Pectorals
- Neck
- Core
- Glutes

ONE-LEGGED BRIDGE
EKA PADA SETU BANDHA SARVANGASANA

PROGRESSION

1 Lie on your back with your arms at your sides, your knees up, and your feet hip-width apart.

2 Push through your feet as you lift your rear off the ground. Keep your arms lengthened.

3 Raise your right leg so that it is at 90 degrees to the ground, with the toes pointing skyward.

4 Hold for 8–10 seconds before returning to the starting position. Repeat with the other leg.

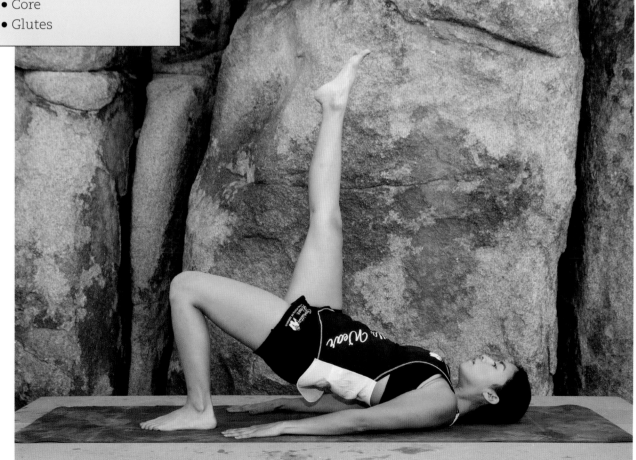

PRIMARY MUSCLE ACTION

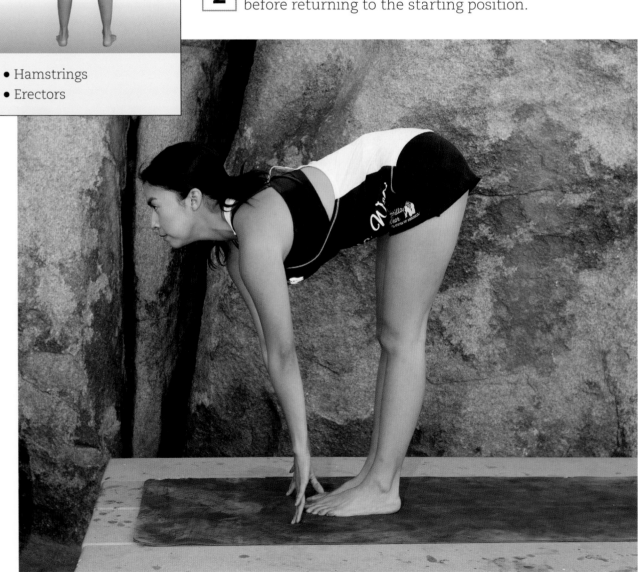

- Hamstrings
- Erectors

HALF-LIFT
ARDHA UTTANASANA

PROGRESSION

1 From a standing position, bend forward while keeping your legs locked, your torso straight, and your back flat. Allow arms and fingers to reach downward so that your fingertips just barely touch the ground.

2 Keep your head up, and hold for 8–10 breaths, before returning to the starting position.

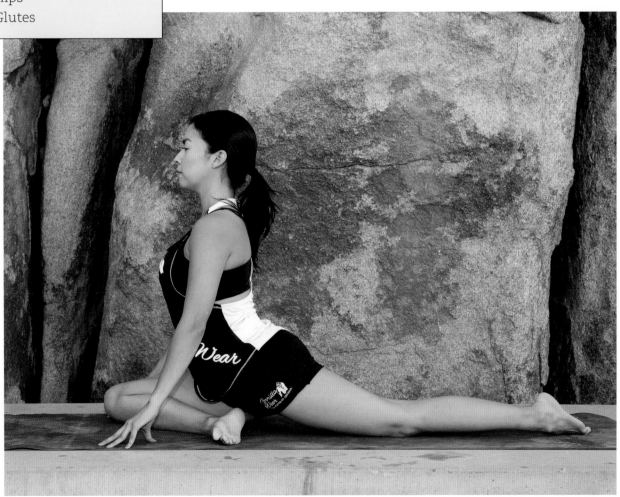

- Hips
- Glutes

HALF-PIGEON
ARDHA KAPOTASANA

PROGRESSION

1 Begin on your hands and knees. Bring your right knee toward your left hand and slide your left foot backward. Bring the right foot through toward the left hip, so that it is in line with the left leg.

2 Keep your fingertips pressed into the ground slightly forward of your hips. Brace your core, and keep your torso and head upright.

3 Hold for 8–10 breaths, then switch sides.

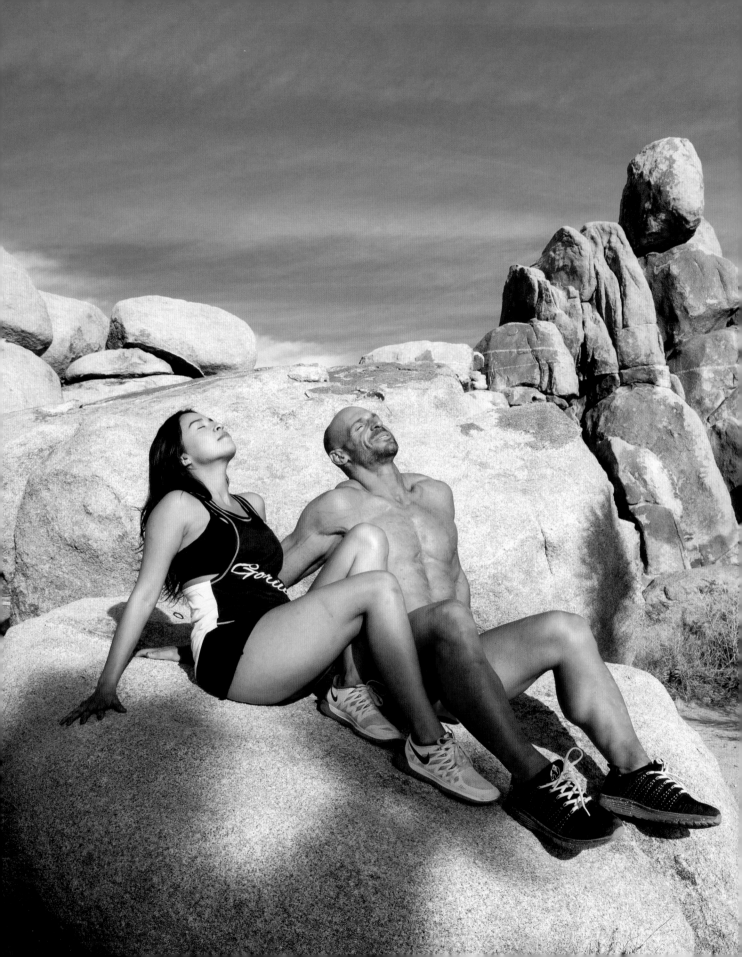

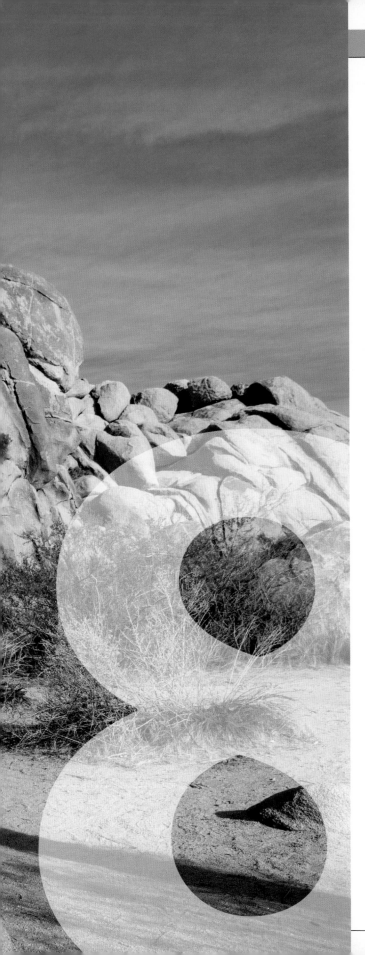

COMING FULL CIRCLE

Congratulations! You've made it through the program. You've cared enough and made time to make *Outdoor Physique* a part of your life, incorporating it into your demanding schedule. Now would be a good time to take some new pictures to compare to the "before" photos you took 12 weeks ago. Of course, photographs don't tell all with regards to your true body transformation, but they sure do say a lot, don't they? Consider also the vast improvements you've made in how you feel and function. I'll bet flights of steps leave you less breathless now, and carrying gallons of paint from your local hardware store is not as taxing. You're probably performing many everyday tasks better than you did before.

For those of you who would now love nothing more than to look at those before pictures but didn't take them at the start of the program, fret not. The fact that this book is even in your hands is a victory in itself. Many do not want a reminder or evidence of their former selves when not at their best, so they neglect to take starting-point pictures. But with social media being what it is, chances are that you have posted some type of before pic somewhere. And if not, then perhaps you were tagged in a photograph in one of your friends' posts. So, you can almost certainly look back and see how far you've come. But your progress is not limited to the physical self in terms of aesthetics. Progress this time around is about so much more. Are you getting around in life with fewer aches and pains? Has your stamina improved over a wide range of activities? How about your posture and the way you carry yourself? Remember, this journey has never been about ripped abs or big arms. Well, actually, at one time it may have been…

My original title for this final part of *Outdoor Physique* was "How the Story Ends." But then I was reminded that the story doesn't end, for it is always evolving into something different, something else. For years, I looked upon the Mr. Olympia physique as the ideal. And I was fortunate in that I was granted access deep into the sport of bodybuilding to see what it was all about. And while a lot of hard work and an entire lifestyle change went into looking like the "physique gods," I realized that not only was it not sustainable over time, it also wasn't the ideal. What

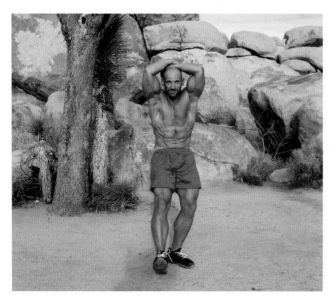

is ideal? That is for each individual to determine, but I can tell you that, for me, now it's about being able to get around comfortably in life, fit into a pair of jeans, and being able to lift, bend, and move a heavy object from point A to point B without hurting myself. Bodybuilding greatness for me has become something so much more important and valuable than a trophy. It means quality of life, and this book is designed to help you put in the work so that you function at or near your best for the long term.

THE JOURNEY CONTINUES

I've always found it interesting when an ending unfolds in a nonfiction book. In fact, even in a fictional story, the story continues in our heads. The characters live on, albeit having experienced change, just as you have, now that you've gone through the *Outdoor Physique* program. However, not only will you pick up this book again and go back to various chapters for reinforcement, but your story never ends.

How could it? That would seem to mean no future change or growth—that everything remains stagnant. And as previously illustrated, growth can come in a variety of ways. A bigger arm or heavier bench press is a limited measure of possible growth. Besides, if that's your goal, you've got the wrong book.

Many of us think the punchline or destination is the end goal. While that is important, the real goal is in the getting there. What is a journey without the, you know, journey? What is a movie without a beginning and middle? What is a song with just the chorus? And when we reach the supposed end, we are really just at a new beginning.

Think about it. Whether celebrating bar mitzvah, taking communion, becoming a Jedi knight, or marking some other graduation or accomplishment, there's always something new to shoot for. One could argue this is drama, which is conflict, and not all conflict is negative. Conflict is what keeps us sharp, on edge, ready for further challenges and betterment.

You might have short-term, daily action goals such as brushing your teeth. And while it may be concluded for that session, the brushing will be repeated later. The brushing of your teeth never ends; it continues throughout your life. That is also the case with fitness. Your daily workout may be concluded, but there is always the next one. And the next workout doesn't always lead to a higher level or an improvement. It certainly can, but it doesn't necessarily need to.

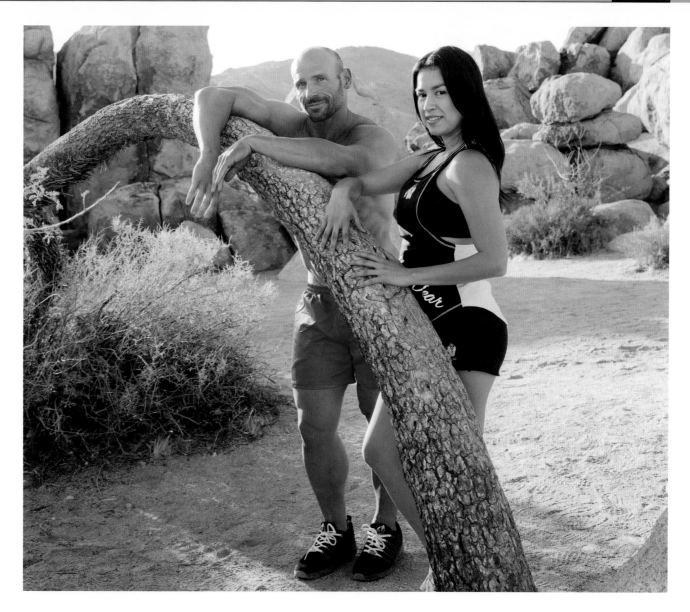

The beautiful thing is that fitness is always there for you, instantly available. Whether it is like a friend you speak to every day or one you pick right up with after no contact for months, exercise is always there, and it never judges or says no. The gym, your portable gym, is like an ever-present well, happy for you to draw from its waters. Drink full, my friends.

THE TRILOGY COMPLETE

This concludes my series of *Physique* transformation books. The first was a plan for getting you to peak fitness for an event. The second was about hitting a mark or goal and staying within striking distance for a lifestyle you could live with. And here we culminate with *Outdoor Physique*, a book about performance and aesthetics, but no gym and no membership fees. Just you. Of course, there are direct correlations between all three volumes in this series. We know that for real results, through a series of angles, focused intensity, proper form, and placing more stress upon working muscle(s), you can do far more with your physique in less time than initially conceived.

Thank you for taking this journey with me. For asking for more. For challenging yourself and for learning and achieving more. Take imperfect action, my friends!

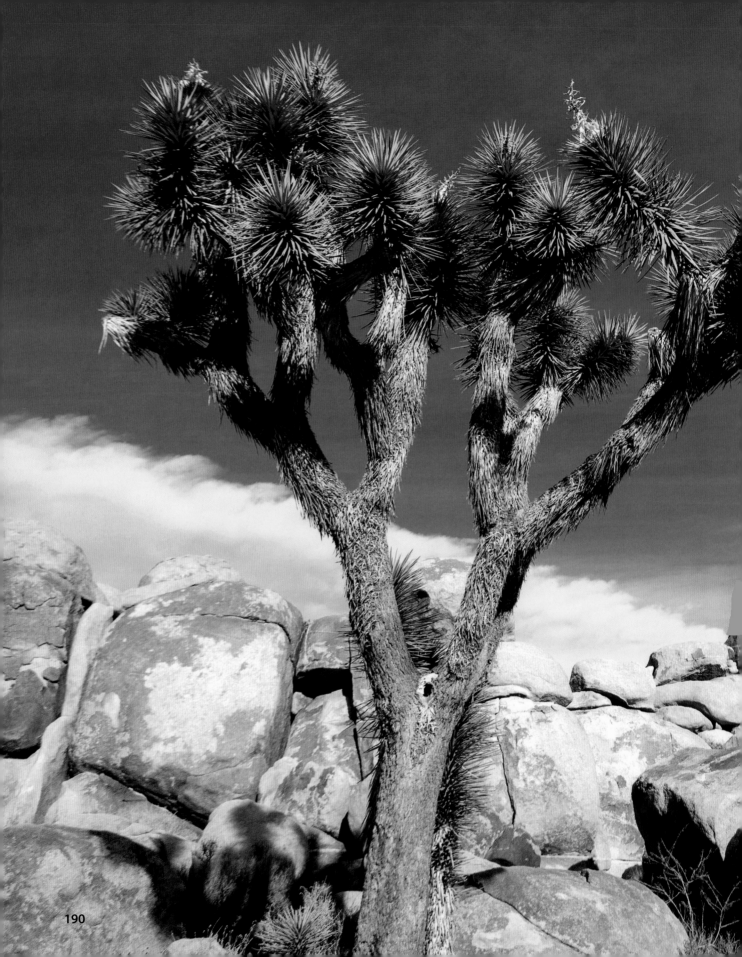

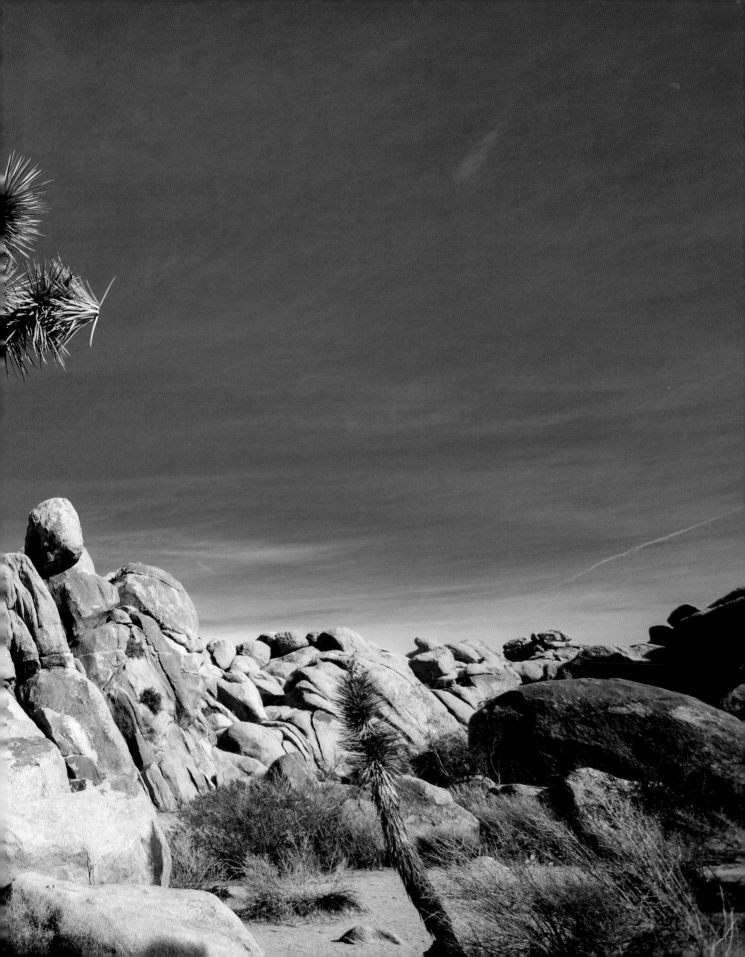

CREDITS

About the Author

Before beginning a career as an internationally published author and personal trainer, Hollis Lance Liebman was a fitness magazine editor, national bodybuilding champion, and physique photographer. He has also served as a bodybuilding and fitness competition judge. Currently a South Carolina resident, Hollis has worked with some of Hollywood's elite, earning himself rave reviews. *Outdoor Physique: Your Portable Body Transformation* is his 13th fitness book. Hollis is also a passionate dog advocate, as evidenced by his popular children's book series *Everyone Loves Lucy*.

Visit hollisliebman.com to keep up to date with all of Hollis's latest news and activities, including fitness tips and complete training programs. Instagram @hllpac

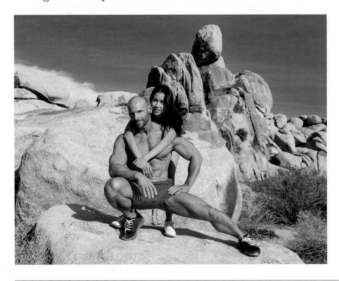

Editorial and design work by Sands Publishing Solutions
sandseditorial.co.uk

Photography by Susan Sheridan
susansheridanphotography.com
Instagram @susansheridanphotography

Model: Daniela Schiller
modalayoga@gmail.com
Instagram @moredaniela_

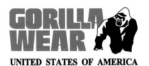

UNITED STATES OF AMERICA

Clothing provided by Gorilla Wear
gorillawear.com
Instagram @gorillawearusa

Additional clothing: Daniela's own

Photographed on location at
Joshua Tree National Park
nps.gov/jotr

ACKNOWLEDGMENTS

The author wishes to thank the national park service at Joshua Tree National Park, Gorilla Wear, and especially the tireless efforts and excellence of David and Sylvia Tombesi-Walton, Simon Murrell, Susan Sheridan, and Daniela Schiller.

This book is dedicated to the memory of my parents, Bruce and Dale Liebman, who indeed made a boy believe he could fly.

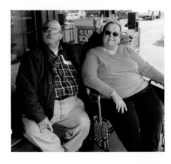